CONTENTS

Chapter 1: Introduction to Learning Disabilities — 1
Chapter 2: Neuroanatomy and Neurodevelopment — 13
Chapter 3: Genetic and Biochemical Factors — 35
Chapter 4: Cognitive and Psychological Mechanisms — 62
Chapter 5: Educational Strategies and Interventions — 96
Chapter 6: Holistic and Complementary Approaches — 120

CHAPTER 1: INTRODUCTION TO LEARNING DISABILITIES

Definition and Scope of Learning Disabilities

Learning disabilities (LDs) are a group of neurological disorders that specifically impair an individual's ability to process, understand, and respond to information in typical ways. These disorders are not indicative of an individual's overall intelligence or potential, but rather affect specific cognitive processes that are crucial for learning. The definition of learning disabilities encompasses a range of challenges including difficulties with reading, writing, mathematics, and other academic skills.

The term "learning disability" is used to describe a significant discrepancy between an individual's expected and actual academic performance, despite having average or above-average intelligence and receiving adequate instruction. These disorders are characterized by specific deficits in processing, such as difficulties in phonological processing, working memory, or executive functioning. For instance, dyslexia involves challenges with accurate and/or fluent word recognition and by poor spelling and decoding abilities. Dysgraphia affects writing abilities, including handwriting and composition. Dyscalculia pertains to difficulties in understanding numbers and mathematical concepts.

Scope and Classification

The scope of learning disabilities is broad and encompasses several distinct categories, each with its own set of characteristics and challenges. The classification of learning disabilities generally falls into the following major categories:

1. **Dyslexia**: This is one of the most well-known learning disabilities, affecting reading skills. Individuals with dyslexia may have difficulties with decoding words, recognizing words, and reading fluently. This can lead to challenges with reading comprehension and spelling.

2. **Dysgraphia**: This refers to difficulties with writing that can manifest as problems with handwriting, spelling, and organizing written expression. Individuals with dysgraphia might struggle with the physical act of writing as well as with written expression and composition.

3. **Dyscalculia**: This involves challenges with mathematical skills, including number sense, calculation, and problem-solving. People with dyscalculia may have difficulties with understanding numerical concepts and performing arithmetic operations.

4. **Nonverbal Learning Disabilities (NVLD)**: This type of learning disability affects nonverbal skills such as spatial awareness, visual-motor coordination, and social interaction. Individuals with NVLD might excel in verbal tasks but struggle with tasks requiring visual-spatial processing and social cues.

Etiology and Causes

The etiology of learning disabilities is multifaceted, involving a combination of genetic, neurological, and environmental factors. Research has shown that learning disabilities can have a hereditary component, suggesting that genetics play a role in their development. For example, dyslexia often runs in families, indicating a genetic predisposition.

Neurological factors also contribute significantly to learning disabilities. Brain imaging studies have identified structural and functional differences in the brains of individuals with learning disabilities. For instance, differences in the areas of the brain responsible for reading and language processing have been observed in individuals with dyslexia. Similarly, studies have shown that deficits in specific neural circuits may underlie difficulties in mathematical processing for those with dyscalculia.

Environmental factors, such as prenatal exposure to toxins, premature birth, or perinatal complications, can also influence the development of learning disabilities. However, learning disabilities are not necessarily caused by poor teaching or lack of educational opportunities; rather, they arise from inherent neurological differences.

Diagnosis and Assessment

Diagnosing learning disabilities involves a comprehensive evaluation that includes a review of the individual's developmental history, educational performance, and cognitive functioning. This typically involves standardized testing to assess various domains such as reading, writing, and mathematics, as well as cognitive abilities including memory, attention, and processing speed.

A diagnosis of a learning disability is usually made by a qualified professional, such as a school psychologist, neuropsychologist, or educational psychologist. The assessment aims to identify specific learning difficulties, rule out other conditions that might affect learning, and determine the extent to which the learning disability affects academic performance.

Impact on Learning and Development

Learning disabilities can have a profound impact on an individual's academic performance and overall development. These challenges can affect self-esteem, motivation, and social interactions. For example, students with learning disabilities might experience frustration and anxiety due to difficulties in keeping up with peers, which can affect their motivation to engage in school and their self-perception.

Despite these challenges, individuals with learning disabilities often have unique strengths and abilities. Many excel in areas that do not rely on their specific areas of difficulty, such as creative thinking, problem-solving, or interpersonal skills. Recognizing and nurturing these strengths is an essential part of supporting individuals with learning disabilities.

Scope of Learning Disabilities

The scope of learning disabilities extends beyond the educational system and affects various aspects of life. Individuals with learning disabilities may encounter challenges in vocational settings, social interactions, and daily living activities. They may require accommodations and supports to succeed in different environments, including workplace adjustments, specialized educational tools, and personal strategies for managing their difficulties.

Conclusion

Learning disabilities are a diverse group of disorders with specific challenges related to processing and understanding information. They are defined by significant discrepancies between expected and actual performance in specific academic areas, despite average or above-average intelligence. The scope of learning disabilities includes various categories such as dyslexia, dysgraphia, dyscalculia, and NVLD, each with its own unique characteristics and impacts. Understanding the definition and scope of learning disabilities is crucial for developing effective interventions and support systems that can help individuals navigate their challenges and achieve their full potential.

Prevalence and Epidemiology

Understanding the prevalence of learning disabilities (LDs) is essential for several reasons, including informing public health strategies, educational practices, and policy-making. The prevalence of learning disabilities varies based on several factors, including the definition and criteria used, the population studied, and regional differences.

In general, research indicates that learning disabilities affect a significant portion of the population. Estimates suggest that approximately 5-15% of school-aged children in developed countries have some form of learning disability. This wide range reflects differences in diagnostic criteria, assessment methods, and cultural contexts.

For instance, dyslexia, one of the most common learning disabilities, affects about 5-10% of the population. Dyscalculia and dysgraphia are less prevalent but still affect a notable percentage of individuals, with estimates ranging from 3-7% for dyscalculia and 5-10% for dysgraphia. Nonverbal learning disabilities (NVLD) are less frequently diagnosed, but estimates suggest that up to 1-3% of individuals may be affected.

Epidemiological Trends

Epidemiological studies provide insights into the distribution and patterns of learning disabilities across different populations. Several factors influence these trends, including age, gender, socioeconomic status, and geographic location.

1. **Age and Developmental Trends**: Learning disabilities are typically identified during the school years, although early signs can be observed in preschool and early childhood. For example, children with dyslexia may exhibit difficulties with language development and early reading skills before formal schooling. As children progress through school, the academic challenges associated with learning disabilities often become more apparent. However, with appropriate interventions and support, some individuals may continue to face challenges into adulthood.

2. **Gender Differences**: Research indicates that learning disabilities are more commonly diagnosed in males than females. For instance, boys are approximately 1.5 to 2 times more likely to be diagnosed with dyslexia compared to girls. The reasons for this gender disparity are not fully understood but may involve biological, psychological, and social factors. Girls may also present with learning disabilities in less overt ways, potentially

leading to underdiagnosis or misdiagnosis.

3. **Socioeconomic Status**: Socioeconomic factors play a significant role in the prevalence and identification of learning disabilities. Children from lower socioeconomic backgrounds may face greater challenges in accessing early screening and intervention services. This can lead to delays in diagnosis and treatment, contributing to disparities in educational outcomes. Additionally, socioeconomic stressors can exacerbate the difficulties associated with learning disabilities.

4. **Geographic and Cultural Variations**: The prevalence of learning disabilities can vary across different geographic regions and cultural contexts. Differences in educational systems, diagnostic practices, and cultural attitudes towards learning disabilities can influence prevalence rates. For example, some countries may have more robust screening programs and early intervention services, leading to higher identification rates of learning disabilities. Conversely, in regions with limited resources or less awareness, learning disabilities may be underreported.

Diagnostic and Reporting Variations

Variations in diagnostic criteria and reporting practices can also impact prevalence estimates. Different countries and organizations use varying definitions and criteria for diagnosing learning disabilities, which can lead to discrepancies in reported prevalence rates. For instance, the criteria used by the American Psychiatric Association in the DSM-5 (Diagnostic and Statistical Manual of Mental Disorders) may differ from those used in other international classifications, such as the ICD-10 (International Classification of Diseases).

Additionally, some learning disabilities may be co-occurring with other conditions, such as attention-deficit/hyperactivity disorder (ADHD) or autism spectrum disorder (ASD), which can complicate diagnosis and affect prevalence estimates. Comorbidity can make it challenging to determine whether difficulties are solely due to a learning disability or if they are part of a broader developmental profile.

Impact on Educational Systems

The prevalence of learning disabilities has significant implications for educational systems. Schools and educators need to be equipped with strategies and resources to identify and support students with learning disabilities. Early intervention and individualized educational plans (IEPs) are crucial for helping students with learning disabilities succeed academically and develop effective coping strategies.

The increasing awareness of learning disabilities has led to improvements in educational practices, including the development of specialized programs, assistive technologies, and targeted interventions. However, there remains a need for ongoing research and advocacy to ensure that all students with learning disabilities receive the support they need.

Public Health and Policy Implications

From a public health perspective, understanding the prevalence of learning disabilities helps in planning and allocating resources for screening, intervention, and support services. Policymakers and educators need to work together to create inclusive educational environments and provide necessary accommodations for students with learning disabilities.

Advocacy and public awareness campaigns are essential for reducing stigma and promoting understanding of learning disabilities. Ensuring that families and educators are informed about the signs and symptoms of learning disabilities can lead to earlier diagnosis and more effective interventions.

Conclusion

The prevalence and epidemiology of learning disabilities reveal that these conditions affect a significant portion of the population, with varying degrees of impact based on age, gender, socioeconomic status, and geographic location. Understanding these patterns helps inform public health strategies, educational practices, and policy-making. Continued research and advocacy are essential for improving diagnosis, intervention, and support for individuals with learning disabilities, ultimately fostering a more inclusive and supportive society.

Diagnostic Criteria and Classification Systems

Accurate diagnosis of learning disabilities (LDs) is crucial for providing effective interventions and support. The diagnostic process involves identifying specific learning difficulties, distinguishing them from other conditions, and ensuring that they significantly impact academic performance. Diagnostic criteria are outlined in several key classification systems, including the DSM-5 (Diagnostic and Statistical Manual of Mental Disorders, Fifth Edition) and the ICD-10/ICD-11 (International Classification of Diseases).

DSM-5 Diagnostic Criteria

The DSM-5, published by the American Psychiatric Association, provides criteria for diagnosing Specific Learning Disorders, which encompass various types of learning disabilities. The criteria include:

1. **Persistent Difficulties**: There must be persistent difficulties in reading, writing, or mathematics, which are significantly below what is expected for the individual's age, education, and level of intelligence. These difficulties must be evident for at least six months despite appropriate instruction.

2. **Impairment in Academic Achievement**: The learning difficulties must result in academic performance that is below expected levels. This impairment must impact the individual's ability to perform well in school or other academic settings.

3. **Exclusion of Other Conditions**: The learning difficulties cannot be better explained by other factors, such as intellectual disabilities, sensory impairments, or

inadequate educational instruction. Additionally, the difficulties must not be attributable to other mental disorders or developmental disorders.

4. **Significant Impact**: The learning difficulties must cause significant interference with academic achievement or daily functioning. This includes difficulties in reading comprehension, written expression, or mathematical reasoning.

Specific learning disorders are further categorized into different types based on the area of difficulty:

- **Dyslexia**: Characterized by difficulties with accurate and/or fluent word recognition and by poor spelling and decoding abilities.
- **Dysgraphia**: Involves difficulties with writing, including handwriting and composition.
- **Dyscalculia**: Refers to difficulties with understanding numbers and mathematical concepts.

ICD-10/ICD-11 Diagnostic Criteria

The ICD-10, published by the World Health Organization (WHO), and its successor, the ICD-11, provide a framework for diagnosing learning disabilities in a global context. The ICD system classifies learning disabilities under the broader category of "Disorders of Intellectual Development" and "Specific Learning Disorders."

1. **ICD-10 Criteria**: The ICD-10 includes learning disorders under the classification of "Specific Developmental Disorders of Scholastic Skills" (F81). This category includes:
    - **Dyslexia**: Difficulty with reading.
    - **Developmental Expressive Language Disorder**: Difficulty with writing and spelling.
    - **Developmental Arithmetic Disorder**: Difficulty with mathematics.

Diagnostic criteria in ICD-10 emphasize:

- Persistent difficulties in one or more areas of academic achievement.
- The difficulties are not due to inadequate instruction, intellectual disability, or other developmental disorders.
- The impairment significantly affects educational or occupational performance.

2. **ICD-11 Criteria**: The ICD-11 provides a more refined classification, incorporating specific learning disorders into the category of "Disorders of Adult Personality and Behavior" (6D00-6D09). This includes:
   - **Dyslexia**: Characterized by difficulties with reading accuracy and fluency.
   - **Developmental Disorder of Mathematical Skills**: Characterized by difficulties with numerical concepts and mathematical reasoning.
   - **Developmental Disorder of Written Expression**: Characterized by difficulties with spelling, handwriting, and written expression.

The ICD-11 criteria are similar to those in the DSM-5, focusing on significant academic impairment and exclusion of other causes.

Classification Systems

In addition to the DSM-5 and ICD systems, other classification frameworks provide insights into learning disabilities:

1. **RTI (Response to Intervention)**: This model is used in educational settings to identify and support students with learning disabilities. RTI involves a tiered approach to intervention, starting with high-quality instruction and increasing levels of support based on student response. If a student does not respond adequately to tiered interventions, further assessment may lead to a formal diagnosis of a learning disability.
2. **WISC-V (Wechsler Intelligence Scale for Children,**

Fifth Edition): This is a widely used cognitive assessment tool that helps in evaluating intellectual functioning and identifying learning disabilities. The WISC-V provides a detailed profile of cognitive strengths and weaknesses, which can be useful in diagnosing specific learning disorders.

3. **Cognitive Processing Models**: Models like the Phonological Processing Model for dyslexia and the Mathematical Processing Model for dyscalculia help in understanding the underlying cognitive processes involved in specific learning disabilities. These models inform the assessment and intervention strategies by focusing on the specific cognitive deficits associated with each type of learning disability.

Diagnostic Challenges

Diagnosing learning disabilities can be challenging due to several factors:

- **Overlap with Other Conditions**: Learning disabilities often co-occur with other conditions, such as ADHD or autism spectrum disorders, making it difficult to isolate specific learning difficulties.
- **Variability in Presentation**: Learning disabilities can present differently across individuals, and symptoms may vary based on age, cognitive development, and educational history.
- **Cultural and Linguistic Factors**: Cultural and linguistic differences can affect the interpretation of diagnostic criteria and the identification of learning disabilities. It is important to consider these factors to avoid misdiagnosis.

Conclusion

The diagnostic criteria and classification systems for learning disabilities provide a structured approach to identifying and understanding these conditions. The DSM-5 and ICD-10/

ICD-11 offer comprehensive frameworks for diagnosing specific learning disorders, while additional models and tools, such as RTI and cognitive processing models, support assessment and intervention. Accurate diagnosis is crucial for providing effective support and interventions, and it requires careful consideration of various factors to ensure a comprehensive understanding of each individual's unique challenges.

CHAPTER 2: NEUROANATOMY AND NEURODEVELOPMENT

Basic Neuroanatomy Relevant to Learning Disabilities

Understanding basic neuroanatomy is crucial for comprehending how learning disabilities (LDs) manifest and are processed in the brain. Learning disabilities often involve specific neural circuits and brain regions that affect cognitive functions essential for learning. This section outlines the key neuroanatomical structures and their roles in learning and how disruptions in these areas can lead to various learning disabilities.

1. Brain Regions Involved in Learning

Cerebral Cortex: The cerebral cortex is the outer layer of the brain and is critical for high-level cognitive functions. It is divided into several lobes, each associated with different aspects of learning:

- **Frontal Lobe**: Involved in executive functions such as planning, decision-making, and problem-solving. It also plays a role in working memory and attention, which are crucial for managing and processing information.
- **Parietal Lobe**: Responsible for integrating sensory information and spatial reasoning. It is involved in mathematical processing and understanding spatial relationships, which are essential for tasks such as arithmetic and geometry.
- **Temporal Lobe**: Associated with auditory processing and language comprehension. It contains structures

like the Wernicke's area, which is important for understanding and producing language. Damage or dysfunction in this area can lead to language-related learning disabilities such as dyslexia.

- **Occipital Lobe**: Primarily responsible for visual processing. This lobe helps in recognizing and interpreting visual information, which is important for reading and visual learning tasks.

Hippocampus: Located within the medial temporal lobe, the hippocampus is crucial for memory formation and consolidation. It helps convert short-term memories into long-term memories, which is vital for learning new information and retaining it over time.

Amygdala: This structure, also located in the temporal lobe, is involved in processing emotions and forming emotional memories. The amygdala interacts with the hippocampus to influence memory based on emotional significance, which can affect learning experiences and emotional responses to academic challenges.

Basal Ganglia: The basal ganglia are a group of nuclei involved in motor control and procedural learning. They play a role in automating skills and habits, such as handwriting. Disruptions in the basal ganglia can affect motor coordination and lead to difficulties with tasks that require fine motor skills, such as those seen in dysgraphia.

2. Neural Pathways and Connectivity

White Matter Tracts: White matter tracts connect different brain regions and facilitate communication between them. Key tracts relevant to learning include:

- **Arcuate Fasciculus**: Connects Broca's area (language production) and Wernicke's area (language comprehension). Disruptions in this pathway can lead to language processing disorders such as dyslexia.
- **Corpus Callosum**: Connects the two hemispheres of

the brain, allowing for coordination between them. Impairments in the corpus callosum can affect tasks that require integration of information from both hemispheres, impacting skills such as reading and writing.

Dorsal and Ventral Streams: These are pathways in the visual system that process different aspects of visual information.

- **Dorsal Stream**: Involved in spatial awareness and visual-motor integration. It helps with tasks such as reading and tracking moving objects.
- **Ventral Stream**: Responsible for object recognition and detailed visual processing. It aids in recognizing letters and words, which is crucial for reading.

3. Neurotransmitter Systems

Dopamine: This neurotransmitter is involved in attention, motivation, and reward processing. Dopamine dysregulation is linked to attention deficits and can impact executive functions. For example, dopamine imbalances are associated with ADHD, which often co-occurs with other learning disabilities.

Serotonin: Plays a role in mood regulation and cognitive functions such as memory and learning. Dysregulation of serotonin levels can affect emotional responses and cognitive processes, potentially influencing learning outcomes.

Glutamate and GABA: These neurotransmitters are involved in excitatory and inhibitory signaling in the brain, respectively. An imbalance between glutamate and GABA can affect synaptic plasticity and learning processes. For instance, excessive glutamatergic activity can lead to neurodevelopmental disorders, while GABAergic dysfunction can impact cognitive control and learning.

4. Brain Plasticity and Learning

Neuroplasticity: Neuroplasticity refers to the brain's ability to reorganize itself by forming new neural connections. This adaptability is crucial for learning and recovery from injury. In individuals with learning disabilities, neuroplasticity can play a role in compensating for deficits and improving learning outcomes through targeted interventions.

Critical Periods: Certain developmental windows are critical for acquiring specific skills, such as language or reading. Disruptions during these periods can lead to learning disabilities. Understanding these critical periods helps in designing effective early interventions to address developmental delays.

5. Impact of Brain Injuries and Developmental Disorders

Developmental Disorders: Conditions such as dyslexia, dysgraphia, and dyscalculia are associated with specific neural circuits and brain regions. For example, dyslexia is linked to abnormalities in the left occipitotemporal cortex, while dysgraphia involves disruptions in the neural pathways responsible for motor control and handwriting.

Acquired Brain Injuries: Injuries to the brain, such as traumatic brain injury (TBI) or stroke, can affect areas involved in learning and cognitive functions. The impact of such injuries on learning can vary depending on the location and severity of the damage.

Conclusion

Basic neuroanatomy provides essential insights into how learning disabilities arise from disruptions in specific brain regions and neural pathways. Understanding the roles of the cerebral cortex, hippocampus, amygdala, basal ganglia, and neurotransmitter systems helps in identifying the underlying mechanisms of learning disabilities. Additionally, knowledge of neuroplasticity and critical periods informs strategies for early intervention and remediation. By exploring these neuroanatomical aspects, researchers and practitioners can develop more effective approaches to diagnosing and supporting individuals with learning disabilities.

Brain Development and Its Impact on Learning

Understanding brain development is crucial for comprehending how learning disabilities arise and affect cognitive functions. The development of the brain influences various aspects of learning, including cognitive skills, emotional regulation, and social interactions. This section outlines the stages of brain development and their impact on learning, highlighting how deviations or disruptions in these processes can lead to learning disabilities.

1. Stages of Brain Development

Prenatal Development: Brain development begins early in prenatal life, with the formation of the neural tube and the development of the central nervous system. Key processes include:

- **Neurogenesis**: The production of neurons occurs during the early stages of fetal development. This process is critical for establishing the basic structure of the brain.
- **Neuronal Migration**: Newly formed neurons migrate to their appropriate locations in the brain, establishing the foundation for neural circuits and brain organization.
- **Synaptogenesis**: The formation of synapses, or connections between neurons, begins in the prenatal period and continues into early postnatal life. Proper synaptogenesis is crucial for effective brain communication and later cognitive functions.

Disruptions during this stage, such as exposure to toxins, genetic abnormalities, or prenatal stress, can impact brain development and increase the risk of learning disabilities.

Early Childhood (0-5 years): This period is marked by rapid brain growth and development, characterized by:

- **Myelination**: The process of forming myelin, a fatty substance that insulates nerve fibers and enhances the speed of neural transmission. Myelination continues through childhood and adolescence and is essential for efficient brain function.
- **Synaptic Pruning**: The process of eliminating excess

synapses to strengthen neural connections that are frequently used. This pruning helps refine neural circuits and optimize brain function. Ineffective pruning can lead to cognitive and learning difficulties.

- **Critical Periods**: Early childhood includes critical periods for acquiring language, motor skills, and sensory processing. For instance, the development of language skills relies on exposure to language during specific developmental windows. Disruptions during these critical periods can result in language and communication disorders.

Middle Childhood (6-12 years): During this stage, the brain continues to mature, with significant developments including:

- **Cognitive and Executive Function Development**: The prefrontal cortex, responsible for executive functions such as planning, attention, and problem-solving, undergoes significant growth. These functions are crucial for academic performance and are often affected in individuals with learning disabilities.

- **Refinement of Neural Networks**: Increased specialization and integration of neural networks support advanced cognitive functions, including reading, writing, and mathematical reasoning. Difficulties in these areas can indicate disruptions in neural network development.

Adolescence (13-18 years): The adolescent brain undergoes important changes that impact learning and behavior:

- **Prefrontal Cortex Maturation**: The prefrontal cortex continues to mature, enhancing abilities related to impulse control, decision-making, and abstract thinking. Delays or abnormalities in this maturation process can affect executive functioning and learning abilities.

- **Increased Synaptic Efficiency**: The brain becomes more efficient in processing information as synaptic connections become stronger and more specialized. This efficiency is crucial for academic achievement and cognitive development.

2. Impact of Brain Development on Learning

Cognitive Skills: Brain development directly impacts cognitive skills essential for learning, such as attention, memory, and problem-solving. For instance:

- **Attention**: The development of attention networks, including the anterior cingulate cortex and the prefrontal cortex, influences the ability to focus and sustain attention. Deficits in these networks can contribute to learning disabilities like ADHD.
- **Memory**: The hippocampus and related structures are crucial for forming and retrieving memories. Impairments in these areas can affect learning and the ability to retain and use information.

Language and Communication: Language development relies on the maturation of areas such as Broca's area and Wernicke's area in the cerebral cortex. Delays or abnormalities in these regions can lead to learning disabilities such as dyslexia and specific language impairments.

Motor Skills: Brain areas involved in motor control, such as the motor cortex and the basal ganglia, impact fine and gross motor skills. Learning disabilities like dysgraphia are associated with disruptions in these motor pathways, affecting handwriting and other written tasks.

Emotional and Social Development: Brain regions such as the amygdala and the prefrontal cortex play roles in emotional regulation and social interactions. Difficulties in these areas can affect behavior and learning, contributing to challenges in social learning environments.

3. Factors Affecting Brain Development

Genetic Factors: Genetic predispositions can influence brain development and the risk of learning disabilities. For example, genetic mutations or variations can affect neural development and function, leading to conditions such as dyslexia or dyscalculia.

Environmental Influences: Environmental factors, including prenatal exposure to toxins, malnutrition, and early life stress, can impact brain development. Positive environments with rich learning experiences support healthy brain development, while adverse conditions can increase the risk of learning difficulties.

Early Intervention: Early intervention programs that provide targeted support during critical periods of development can mitigate the impact of learning disabilities. For example, early literacy programs can help address delays in reading and language skills.

4. Neuroplasticity and Learning

Neuroplasticity: The brain's ability to reorganize and form new connections is essential for learning and adaptation. Neuroplasticity allows individuals with learning disabilities to develop compensatory strategies and improve their skills through targeted interventions.

Compensatory Mechanisms: Individuals with learning disabilities may rely on alternative cognitive strategies or neural pathways to compensate for their difficulties. Understanding these compensatory mechanisms can help tailor interventions to support effective learning.

Conclusion

Brain development plays a critical role in shaping learning abilities and the manifestation of learning disabilities. From prenatal development through adolescence, various stages of brain growth impact cognitive, language, motor, and emotional skills essential for learning. Factors such as genetics, environment, and early intervention influence brain development and learning outcomes. By understanding these developmental processes and their impact on learning, educators, clinicians, and researchers can develop effective strategies to support individuals with learning disabilities and enhance their educational experiences.

Structural Abnormalities and Functional Dysregulation

Structural abnormalities and functional dysregulation in the brain can significantly impact cognitive processes and contribute to learning disabilities (LDs). Understanding these disruptions is crucial for diagnosing, treating, and developing targeted interventions for various learning disabilities. This section explores common structural abnormalities and functional dysregulation associated with learning disabilities, providing insights into their implications for learning and behavior.

1. Structural Abnormalities

Cortical Dysplasia: Cortical dysplasia refers to abnormal development of the cerebral cortex, which can affect its organization and function. This condition can lead to difficulties in learning and cognitive functions, including problems with language, attention, and motor skills. Abnormalities in cortical development are often seen in conditions such as epilepsy, which can also impact learning.

Hippocampal Abnormalities: The hippocampus, crucial for memory formation and spatial navigation, can exhibit abnormalities in conditions like dyslexia and specific learning disabilities. Structural changes in the hippocampus, such as reduced volume or altered connectivity, can affect memory consolidation and retrieval, leading to difficulties in learning and academic performance.

Basal Ganglia Disruptions: The basal ganglia are involved in motor control and procedural learning. Structural abnormalities in the basal ganglia can contribute to learning disabilities such as dysgraphia, where difficulties with handwriting and fine motor skills are evident. Structural disruptions may also affect the ability to automate skills and coordinate motor tasks.

Corpus Callosum Abnormalities: The corpus callosum connects the left and right hemispheres of the brain, facilitating communication between them. Abnormalities in the corpus callosum, such as reduced size or agenesis (absence of the corpus callosum), can impact tasks requiring bilateral coordination and integration of information from both hemispheres. This can contribute to difficulties in reading, writing, and complex problem-solving.

Gray Matter and White Matter Abnormalities: Gray matter contains neuronal cell bodies, while white matter consists of myelinated axons connecting different brain regions. Abnormalities in gray matter volume or white matter integrity can affect cognitive functions and learning. For example, reduced gray matter in the left temporo-parietal region has been associated with dyslexia, while white matter abnormalities in the frontal and parietal regions can impact executive functions and attention.

2. Functional Dysregulation

Dysregulation of the Prefrontal Cortex: The prefrontal cortex is involved in executive functions such as planning, working memory, and decision-making. Functional dysregulation in this area can lead to difficulties with attention, organization, and problem-solving, contributing to learning disabilities like ADHD. Functional imaging studies often reveal reduced activation or connectivity in the prefrontal cortex in individuals with executive function deficits.

Language Processing Disruptions: Functional dysregulation in regions involved in language processing, such as Broca's area and Wernicke's area, can affect reading and language comprehension. In dyslexia, for instance, functional imaging studies show reduced activation in the left temporo-parietal cortex during reading tasks, indicating impaired language processing.

Visual Processing Abnormalities: The occipital lobe, responsible for visual processing, can exhibit functional dysregulation in individuals with learning disabilities related to visual perception, such as dyslexia. Functional imaging studies may reveal altered activation patterns in the visual processing areas, impacting reading and visual recognition abilities.

Attention and Working Memory: Functional dysregulation in brain networks responsible for attention and working memory, such as the fronto-parietal network, can affect learning. Individuals with ADHD, for example, often show altered activation in brain regions involved in sustaining attention and managing working memory tasks.

Emotional and Behavioral Regulation: Functional dysregulation in the amygdala and prefrontal cortex can impact emotional regulation and behavior, which can, in turn, affect learning. Individuals with learning disabilities may experience heightened emotional responses or difficulties with behavioral control, influencing their ability to engage in learning tasks.

3. Neuroimaging Findings

Magnetic Resonance Imaging (MRI): MRI is used to identify structural abnormalities in the brain. For example, MRI can reveal cortical thickness, hippocampal volume, and white matter integrity, providing insights into structural changes associated with learning disabilities.

Functional MRI (fMRI): fMRI measures brain activity by detecting changes in blood flow. It helps identify functional dysregulation by revealing patterns of brain activation during cognitive tasks. fMRI studies have shown altered activation in brain regions involved in language, attention, and executive functions in individuals with learning disabilities.

Diffusion Tensor Imaging (DTI): DTI is used to assess white matter integrity by measuring the diffusion of water molecules in the brain. It can identify disruptions in white matter tracts, providing insights into the connectivity and communication between brain regions in individuals with learning disabilities.

4. Genetic and Environmental Influences

Genetic Factors: Genetic predispositions can influence structural and functional abnormalities in the brain. Research into gene-environment interactions helps to identify genetic markers associated with learning disabilities, such as dyslexia or dyscalculia.

Environmental Factors: Prenatal and early life experiences, including exposure to toxins, malnutrition, and stress, can impact brain development and contribute to structural and functional dysregulation. Early interventions and positive environmental factors can help mitigate these impacts and support healthy brain development.

5. Implications for Intervention and Support

Targeted Interventions: Understanding structural abnormalities and functional dysregulation helps in developing targeted interventions for individuals with learning disabilities. For example, interventions focusing on specific cognitive skills, such as language processing or executive functions, can address the underlying neuroanatomical and functional issues.

Neuroplasticity and Remediation: Neuroplasticity, the brain's ability to reorganize and adapt, plays a role in remediation and rehabilitation. Interventions that leverage neuroplasticity, such as cognitive training and specialized educational approaches, can help individuals develop compensatory strategies and improve learning outcomes.

Conclusion

Structural abnormalities and functional dysregulation in the brain are key factors contributing to learning disabilities. By understanding the specific brain regions and networks involved, as well as the impact of genetic and environmental influences, researchers and clinicians can develop more effective diagnostic and therapeutic approaches. Neuroimaging techniques provide valuable insights into these disruptions, guiding targeted interventions and support strategies to enhance learning and academic achievement.

Neuroplasticity and Learning Processes

Neuroplasticity, the brain's ability to reorganize itself by forming new neural connections, is a fundamental concept in understanding learning and adaptation. This section explores how neuroplasticity underpins learning processes, its implications for learning disabilities, and the ways in which targeted interventions can harness neuroplasticity to improve learning outcomes.

1. Understanding Neuroplasticity

Types of Neuroplasticity

- **Structural Plasticity**: Refers to changes in the brain's physical structure in response to learning and experience. This includes alterations in dendritic spines, synapse formation, and changes in gray and white matter volume. Structural plasticity allows for the creation of new neural circuits and the strengthening of existing ones.

- **Functional Plasticity**: Involves changes in the brain's functional organization. This type of plasticity enables different brain regions to take over functions previously performed by damaged or less active areas. Functional plasticity is critical for recovering lost skills and adapting to new learning demands.

Mechanisms of Neuroplasticity

- **Synaptic Plasticity**: Changes in the strength and efficacy of synaptic connections between neurons. Key processes include long-term potentiation (LTP) and long-term depression (LTD), which modulate synaptic strength based on experience and learning.

- **Neurogenesis**: The formation of new neurons from neural stem cells. Although more prominent during development, neurogenesis can occur in specific brain regions such as the hippocampus throughout life, contributing to learning and memory.

- **Myelination**: The process of forming a myelin sheath around axons to increase the speed and efficiency of neural transmission. Myelination can be influenced by learning and experience, enhancing cognitive functions and motor skills.

2. Neuroplasticity and Learning

Learning and Memory Formation

- **Skill Acquisition**: Neuroplasticity facilitates the acquisition of new skills by modifying existing neural circuits and forming new ones. Repeated practice and exposure lead to strengthened connections and increased efficiency in the relevant brain regions.
- **Memory Consolidation**: The process of stabilizing and integrating new information into long-term memory. Neuroplasticity supports memory consolidation by reorganizing neural circuits and strengthening synaptic connections involved in storing and retrieving information.

Adaptation to New Experiences

- **Cognitive Flexibility**: The brain's ability to adapt to new information and changing conditions. Neuroplasticity supports cognitive flexibility by allowing the brain to reorganize and optimize neural pathways in response to novel experiences and challenges.
- **Compensation for Injury or Damage**: When specific brain areas are damaged, neuroplasticity allows other regions to compensate for lost functions. For example, following a stroke, other parts of the brain may take over tasks previously managed by the affected areas.

3. Neuroplasticity and Learning Disabilities

Impact of Learning Disabilities on Neuroplasticity

- **Reduced Plasticity**: Learning disabilities can be associated with reduced neuroplasticity in certain brain regions, impacting the ability to acquire and integrate new skills. For instance, dyslexia may involve reduced plasticity in areas related to language processing.

- **Compensatory Mechanisms**: Individuals with learning disabilities often develop alternative strategies or rely on different neural circuits to compensate for their difficulties. Understanding these compensatory mechanisms can inform the development of targeted interventions.

Interventions to Enhance Neuroplasticity

- **Cognitive Training**: Structured cognitive training programs aim to enhance specific cognitive functions by stimulating neuroplasticity. For example, working memory training can improve attention and executive functions in individuals with ADHD.

- **Educational Strategies**: Evidence-based educational interventions, such as multisensory approaches and differentiated instruction, can support neuroplasticity by providing alternative learning pathways and reinforcing neural connections related to academic skills.

- **Assistive Technologies**: Tools such as speech-to-text software, audiobooks, and educational apps can help individuals with learning disabilities engage with content in ways that support neuroplasticity and facilitate learning.

4. Factors Influencing Neuroplasticity

Age and Developmental Stage

- **Critical Periods**: Certain periods in development are characterized by heightened neuroplasticity, allowing for rapid learning and acquisition of specific skills. For example, early childhood is a critical period for language acquisition.

- **Lifelong Plasticity**: Although plasticity is more pronounced during development, the adult brain retains the capacity for neuroplastic changes in response to learning and experience.

Environmental Enrichment

- **Stimulating Environments**: Environments rich in stimuli and learning opportunities can enhance neuroplasticity by promoting neural growth and connectivity. Enrichment can include educational activities, social interactions, and physical exercise.
- **Stress and Adversity**: Chronic stress and adverse experiences can negatively impact neuroplasticity and learning. Stress can alter brain function and structure, potentially leading to difficulties in learning and cognitive performance.

5. Implications for Educational and Clinical Practice

Personalized Learning Approaches

- **Individualized Instruction**: Tailoring educational strategies to meet the specific needs of learners with learning disabilities can optimize neuroplasticity and support skill development. Personalized approaches consider each individual's strengths and challenges.
- **Early Intervention**: Early identification and intervention can leverage neuroplasticity to address learning difficulties before they become entrenched. Early support can help maximize the brain's capacity for adaptation and learning.

Supportive Environments

- **Inclusive Education**: Creating inclusive educational environments that accommodate diverse learning needs can foster neuroplasticity by providing varied learning experiences and support.
- **Family and Community Involvement**: Engaging families and communities in supporting learning and

development can enhance neuroplasticity by creating a supportive network for individuals with learning disabilities.

Conclusion

Neuroplasticity is a fundamental process underlying learning and adaptation. By understanding how neuroplasticity facilitates skill acquisition, memory formation, and adaptation to new experiences, researchers and practitioners can better address learning disabilities and develop effective interventions. Targeted cognitive training, educational strategies, and supportive environments harness the power of neuroplasticity to improve learning outcomes and support individuals with learning disabilities.

Neuroimaging Techniques and Findings

Neuroimaging techniques are pivotal in understanding the brain's structure and function, especially in the context of learning disabilities. These techniques provide detailed insights into brain abnormalities, functional dysregulation, and the underlying neurobiological mechanisms of various learning disabilities. This section discusses the major neuroimaging methods, their applications, and the findings relevant to learning disabilities.

1. Types of Neuroimaging Techniques

Structural Magnetic Resonance Imaging (MRI)

- **Description**: Structural MRI provides detailed images of brain anatomy by measuring the distribution of water molecules in brain tissues. It is particularly useful for examining brain structures, detecting abnormalities, and assessing brain volume.
- **Applications**: Structural MRI is used to identify anatomical abnormalities associated with learning disabilities. For example:
  - **Dyslexia**: Structural MRI studies have found

reduced volume in the left temporo-parietal cortex, an area involved in language processing.
- **Dysgraphia**: Abnormalities in the motor cortex and basal ganglia have been observed, impacting handwriting and fine motor skills.
- **ADHD**: Structural MRI has revealed differences in the size and shape of the prefrontal cortex and basal ganglia, affecting attention and executive functions.

Functional Magnetic Resonance Imaging (fMRI)

- **Description**: fMRI measures brain activity by detecting changes in blood flow and oxygenation levels associated with neural activity. It provides insights into brain function and how different brain regions interact during cognitive tasks.
- **Applications**: fMRI is used to investigate functional dysregulation in learning disabilities. For instance:
  - **Dyslexia**: fMRI studies show reduced activation in the left inferior frontal gyrus and the superior temporal gyrus during reading tasks, indicating difficulties in language processing.
  - **ADHD**: Functional imaging reveals altered activation patterns in the prefrontal cortex and striatum during tasks requiring attention and impulse control.
  - **Autism Spectrum Disorder (ASD)**: Abnormal connectivity and activation patterns in social and communication networks are observed.

Diffusion Tensor Imaging (DTI)

- **Description**: DTI is an MRI-based technique that measures the diffusion of water molecules along white matter tracts, providing information about the integrity and organization of white matter pathways.
- **Applications**: DTI is used to assess white matter abnormalities related to learning disabilities. For

example:
- **Dyslexia**: DTI studies have shown reduced fractional anisotropy in the left arcuate fasciculus, a key pathway for language and reading.
- **ADHD**: Altered white matter connectivity in the prefrontal cortex and corpus callosum has been observed, affecting attention and executive functions.
- **Specific Learning Disabilities**: DTI findings indicate disrupted white matter tracts in regions related to motor control and spatial reasoning.

Electroencephalography (EEG)

- **Description**: EEG records electrical activity along the scalp, providing real-time data on brain wave patterns and their variations. It is useful for assessing neural activity and timing of cognitive processes.
- **Applications**: EEG is employed to study neural oscillations and event-related potentials associated with learning disabilities. For example:
  - **ADHD**: EEG studies often reveal atypical theta/beta ratios and altered event-related potentials during attention tasks.
  - **Dyslexia**: EEG research indicates differences in neural processing during reading and phonological tasks, with variations in N400 and P300 components.

Magnetoencephalography (MEG)

- **Description**: MEG measures the magnetic fields generated by neural activity, offering high temporal resolution and spatial localization of brain function.
- **Applications**: MEG is used to explore dynamic brain activity related to learning disabilities. For instance:
  - **Dyslexia**: MEG studies reveal abnormal

activation patterns in the left hemisphere during language processing tasks.
- **ADHD**: Altered oscillatory activity and connectivity patterns in brain networks related to attention and executive functions are observed.

2. Findings Relevant to Learning Disabilities

Dyslexia

- **Structural Findings**: Reduced gray matter volume in the left posterior superior temporal gyrus and abnormalities in the planum temporale.
- **Functional Findings**: Decreased activation in the left inferior frontal gyrus and the superior temporal gyrus during reading tasks.
- **Connectivity Findings**: Disrupted connectivity in the arcuate fasciculus and other language-related pathways.

ADHD

- **Structural Findings**: Smaller volumes of the prefrontal cortex, basal ganglia, and cerebellum.
- **Functional Findings**: Altered activation in the prefrontal cortex and striatum, particularly during tasks requiring attention and impulse control.
- **Connectivity Findings**: Abnormal connectivity in fronto-parietal and default mode networks, affecting cognitive control and attention.

Dysgraphia

- **Structural Findings**: Abnormalities in the motor cortex and basal ganglia, impacting motor coordination and handwriting.
- **Functional Findings**: Reduced activation in the left motor cortex and supplementary motor area during writing tasks.

- **Connectivity Findings**: Disrupted connectivity between motor and language regions, affecting motor planning and execution.

Autism Spectrum Disorder (ASD)

- **Structural Findings**: Enlarged lateral ventricles, reduced gray matter in areas related to social processing, and atypical development of the corpus callosum.
- **Functional Findings**: Abnormal activation in social cognition networks, including the amygdala and superior temporal sulcus.
- **Connectivity Findings**: Altered connectivity in the default mode network and between social and communication regions.

3. Implications for Diagnosis and Intervention

Early Diagnosis

- Neuroimaging provides critical insights into the neurobiological underpinnings of learning disabilities, enabling early diagnosis and intervention. Early identification of structural and functional abnormalities can facilitate timely and targeted therapeutic approaches.

Targeted Interventions

- Neuroimaging findings inform the development of personalized interventions by highlighting specific brain regions and networks involved in learning disabilities. For example, targeted cognitive training and educational strategies can be designed to address identified neural deficits.

Monitoring Progress

- Neuroimaging techniques can be used to monitor changes in brain structure and function over time, assessing the effectiveness of interventions and guiding adjustments to treatment plans.

Conclusion

Neuroimaging techniques are invaluable tools for exploring the brain's structure and function in the context of learning disabilities. By providing detailed insights into anatomical abnormalities, functional dysregulation, and connectivity patterns, neuroimaging helps advance our understanding of learning disabilities and informs the development of effective diagnostic and therapeutic approaches. As technology continues to evolve, neuroimaging will play an increasingly critical role in optimizing educational and clinical practices for individuals with learning disabilities.

CHAPTER 3: GENETIC AND BIOCHEMICAL FACTORS

Genetic Basis of Learning Disabilities

The genetic basis of learning disabilities involves understanding how genetic factors contribute to the development and manifestation of these conditions. Learning disabilities, including dyslexia, dyscalculia, and ADHD, have been shown to have a hereditary component, suggesting that genetics play a significant role in their etiology. This section delves into the genetic underpinnings of learning disabilities, exploring specific genes, genetic variants, and the interaction between genetic and environmental factors.

1. Overview of Genetic Contributions

Heritability of Learning Disabilities

- **Dyslexia**: Studies have demonstrated that dyslexia has a substantial heritable component, with estimates suggesting that around 40-60% of the variance in dyslexia risk can be attributed to genetic factors. Family and twin studies have consistently shown that dyslexia tends to run in families.
- **ADHD**: The heritability of ADHD is estimated to be around 70-80%, indicating a strong genetic influence. Twin studies reveal that if one twin has ADHD, the likelihood of the other twin also having the disorder is significantly higher.

- **Dyscalculia**: Research suggests a heritable component in dyscalculia, though less well-studied than dyslexia and ADHD. Twin studies indicate that genetic factors contribute to individual differences in mathematical abilities.

Genetic Studies and Approaches

- **Linkage Studies**: Linkage studies investigate the co-occurrence of learning disabilities with specific genetic markers across families. These studies have identified potential chromosomal regions linked to dyslexia (e.g., chromosomes 6p21, 15q21) and ADHD (e.g., chromosomes 5, 16).
- **Association Studies**: Association studies examine correlations between specific genetic variants and learning disabilities. For example, polymorphisms in genes such as the DYX1C1 gene (linked to dyslexia) and the DRD4 gene (associated with ADHD) have been identified.
- **Genome-Wide Association Studies (GWAS)**: GWAS involve scanning the entire genome for genetic variants associated with learning disabilities. Recent GWAS have identified several risk loci for dyslexia and ADHD, revealing complex genetic architectures involving multiple genes with small effects.

2. Specific Genes and Genetic Variants

Dyslexia

- **DYX1C1**: This gene is associated with dyslexia and is involved in neuronal migration and brain development. Variants in DYX1C1 are thought to impact reading abilities by affecting the formation and function of brain circuits related to language.
- **ROBO1**: The ROBO1 gene is implicated in dyslexia and is involved in the development of neural pathways.

Variants in ROBO1 can influence the connectivity of brain regions responsible for language processing.

- **KIAA0319**: This gene is associated with dyslexia and is involved in brain development and function. Variants in KIAA0319 have been linked to differences in reading abilities and phonological processing.

ADHD

- **DRD4**: The DRD4 gene encodes a dopamine receptor and has been associated with ADHD. Variants in DRD4 are thought to influence dopamine regulation, which impacts attention and impulse control.
- **DAT1**: The DAT1 gene encodes the dopamine transporter and is linked to ADHD. Variants in DAT1 can affect dopamine reuptake, influencing attention and hyperactivity.
- **SNAP-25**: The SNAP-25 gene is involved in synaptic neurotransmitter release. Variants in SNAP-25 have been associated with ADHD, affecting neurotransmission and cognitive functions.

Dyscalculia

- **ATP2A2**: The ATP2A2 gene, involved in calcium signaling and neuronal function, has been linked to dyscalculia. Variants in ATP2A2 may affect mathematical processing and numerical abilities.
- **GRIN2A**: The GRIN2A gene encodes a subunit of the NMDA receptor, which is involved in synaptic plasticity. Variants in GRIN2A have been associated with mathematical learning difficulties.

3. Gene-Environment Interactions

Epigenetics

- **Definition**: Epigenetics refers to changes in gene expression that do not involve alterations to the

DNA sequence. Environmental factors can influence epigenetic modifications, impacting the risk and severity of learning disabilities.

- **Impact**: Epigenetic changes can affect genes involved in brain development and function. For instance, exposure to prenatal stress or toxins may lead to epigenetic modifications that influence the development of learning disabilities.

Gene-Environment Interaction

- **Example**: Interaction between genetic predisposition and environmental factors can modify the risk of developing learning disabilities. For example, a child with a genetic predisposition to dyslexia may be more likely to exhibit reading difficulties if exposed to adverse educational environments.

- **Research**: Studies exploring gene-environment interactions provide insights into how genetic risk factors are modulated by environmental influences. This research can inform preventive strategies and interventions tailored to individuals' genetic and environmental contexts.

4. Implications for Diagnosis and Treatment

Genetic Screening

- **Application**: Genetic screening for learning disabilities is an emerging area of research. Identifying specific genetic variants associated with learning disabilities can facilitate early diagnosis and personalized interventions.

- **Ethical Considerations**: The use of genetic information raises ethical questions about privacy, potential stigmatization, and the implications of genetic findings for individuals and families.

Personalized Interventions

- **Targeted Approaches**: Understanding the genetic basis of learning disabilities allows for the development of targeted interventions. Personalized educational strategies and therapies can be designed based on individuals' genetic profiles and specific needs.

- **Future Directions**: Advances in genetic research and technology hold promise for improving the accuracy of diagnosis and the effectiveness of interventions. Continued research into the genetic basis of learning disabilities will enhance our ability to support individuals and optimize educational outcomes.

Conclusion

The genetic basis of learning disabilities reveals a complex interplay of genetic variants and their impact on brain function and development. By identifying specific genes and genetic variants associated with learning disabilities, researchers and clinicians can gain valuable insights into the underlying mechanisms and develop targeted interventions. Understanding gene-environment interactions and incorporating genetic information into diagnostic and therapeutic approaches will further enhance our ability to support individuals with learning disabilities and improve their educational experiences.

Molecular Genetics and Gene-Environment Interactions

Molecular genetics and gene-environment interactions play a crucial role in understanding the development and manifestation of learning disabilities. By examining how genetic factors influence susceptibility to learning disabilities and how environmental factors modify these genetic risks, researchers can gain insights into the complex interplay between genetics and the environment. This section explores the molecular genetics underlying learning disabilities and the ways in which environmental factors can interact with genetic predispositions.

1. Molecular Genetics of Learning Disabilities

Genetic Variants and Learning Disabilities

- **Single Nucleotide Polymorphisms (SNPs)**: SNPs are variations at a single nucleotide position in the DNA sequence among individuals. Certain SNPs have been associated with learning disabilities. For instance:
    - **Dyslexia**: SNPs in genes such as DYX1C1, KIAA0319, and ROBO1 have been linked to dyslexia. These variants are involved in brain development and function, impacting language processing and reading abilities.
    - **ADHD**: SNPs in genes such as DRD4, DAT1, and SNAP-25 have been associated with ADHD. These variants affect neurotransmitter systems, influencing attention, impulse control, and executive functions.
    - **Dyscalculia**: SNPs in genes like ATP2A2 and GRIN2A are linked to dyscalculia, affecting mathematical processing and numerical abilities.
- **Copy Number Variations (CNVs)**: CNVs involve deletions or duplications of large DNA segments. CNVs can impact gene dosage and function, influencing learning disabilities. For example:
    - **Autism Spectrum Disorder (ASD)**: CNVs in genes such as 16p11.2 have been associated with ASD, affecting brain development and function related to social and communication skills.

Gene Expression and Regulation

- **Transcription Factors**: Transcription factors regulate the expression of genes involved in brain development and function. Variants in transcription factors can influence learning disabilities by altering gene expression patterns. For example, mutations in the FOXP2 gene, a transcription factor involved in speech and language development, are linked to speech and language disorders.

- **Epigenetic Modifications**: Epigenetic modifications, such as DNA methylation and histone modification, regulate gene expression without altering the DNA sequence. Epigenetic changes can affect genes involved in learning and memory. For instance, stress and environmental factors can lead to epigenetic modifications that impact cognitive functions and increase susceptibility to learning disabilities.

2. Gene-Environment Interactions

Influence of Environmental Factors on Genetic Risk

- **Prenatal Environment**: Environmental factors during pregnancy, such as maternal nutrition, stress, and exposure to toxins, can interact with genetic predispositions to influence the risk of learning disabilities. For example:
    - **Dyslexia**: Prenatal exposure to high levels of stress or toxins can interact with genetic risk factors for dyslexia, potentially exacerbating reading difficulties.
    - **ADHD**: Prenatal exposure to nicotine or alcohol may interact with genetic risk factors for ADHD, increasing the likelihood of developing attention and impulse control issues.
- **Early Childhood Environment**: Early life experiences, including educational opportunities, social interactions, and parental involvement, can modify genetic risks for learning disabilities. For example:
    - **Dysgraphia**: Early educational interventions and support can help mitigate the impact of genetic risk factors for dysgraphia by providing targeted skill development.
    - **Dyscalculia**: Exposure to enriched learning environments and early mathematical experiences can influence the expression of

genetic risk factors for dyscalculia.

Gene-Environment Interaction Mechanisms

- **Neurodevelopmental Pathways**: Gene-environment interactions can affect neurodevelopmental pathways critical for learning. For example:
    - **Dyslexia**: Genetic variants associated with dyslexia may interact with environmental factors to influence the development of neural circuits involved in reading and language processing.
    - **ADHD**: Gene-environment interactions can impact neurotransmitter systems and brain networks involved in attention and executive functions.
- **Plasticity and Adaptation**: The brain's plasticity allows for adaptation to environmental influences. Gene-environment interactions can shape neural development and function, affecting learning outcomes. For example:
    - **Autism Spectrum Disorder (ASD)**: Gene-environment interactions can influence the development of social and communication skills in ASD. Early intervention and supportive environments can enhance plasticity and improve outcomes.

3. Implications for Research and Practice

Understanding Complex Interactions

- **Integrated Approaches**: Research integrating genetic, epigenetic, and environmental factors provides a comprehensive understanding of learning disabilities. Identifying specific gene-environment interactions helps elucidate the mechanisms underlying these conditions.
- **Personalized Interventions**: Knowledge of gene-environment interactions can inform personalized

interventions. Tailoring educational and therapeutic strategies based on genetic and environmental factors can improve effectiveness and outcomes.

Preventive and Remedial Strategies

- **Early Identification**: Identifying genetic and environmental risk factors early can facilitate preventive measures and early interventions. For example, monitoring prenatal and early childhood environments can help identify at-risk individuals and provide timely support.
- **Environmental Modifications**: Creating supportive and enriched environments can mitigate the impact of genetic risk factors. Educational programs, parental support, and community resources can enhance learning and development for individuals with learning disabilities.

4. Future Directions

Advancements in Genomic Research

- **Genome-Wide Studies**: Advances in genomic research, such as whole-genome sequencing and epigenetic analyses, will provide deeper insights into the genetic and environmental factors influencing learning disabilities.
- **Longitudinal Studies**: Longitudinal studies tracking genetic and environmental factors over time will improve understanding of how gene-environment interactions influence the development and progression of learning disabilities.

Translational Research

- **Clinical Applications**: Translating research findings into clinical practice will enhance diagnostic accuracy and intervention strategies. Incorporating genetic and environmental information into clinical assessments

will improve personalized care for individuals with learning disabilities.
- **Policy and Education**: Research on gene-environment interactions can inform policies and educational practices aimed at supporting individuals with learning disabilities and promoting equitable access to resources and interventions.

Conclusion

Molecular genetics and gene-environment interactions provide critical insights into the development and manifestation of learning disabilities. By understanding how genetic factors and environmental influences interact, researchers and clinicians can develop more effective diagnostic and therapeutic approaches. Advances in genetic research, along with a focus on personalized interventions and supportive environments, will enhance our ability to address learning disabilities and improve outcomes for affected individuals.

Neurotransmitter Systems and Their Role

Neurotransmitter systems are crucial for understanding the neurobiological underpinnings of learning disabilities. Neurotransmitters are chemical messengers that transmit signals across synapses, facilitating communication between neurons. Dysregulation of these systems can affect cognitive functions and contribute to various learning disabilities, including dyslexia, ADHD, and dyscalculia. This section explores the major neurotransmitter systems involved in learning disabilities, their roles in brain function, and how their dysfunction can impact learning and behavior.

1. Overview of Major Neurotransmitter Systems

Dopaminergic System

- **Function**: The dopaminergic system involves dopamine

(DA), a neurotransmitter that plays a key role in reward, motivation, attention, and executive functions. Dopamine pathways include the mesolimbic, mesocortical, and nigrostriatal systems.

- **Role in Learning Disabilities**:
    - **ADHD**: Dysregulation of dopamine pathways, particularly in the prefrontal cortex and striatum, is associated with ADHD. Alterations in dopamine receptor density and dopamine transporter function can affect attention, impulse control, and executive functions.
    - **Dyslexia**: Research suggests that dopamine system abnormalities may influence reading difficulties by affecting cognitive control and processing speed.

Noradrenergic System

- **Function**: The noradrenergic system involves norepinephrine (NE), which is crucial for arousal, attention, and stress responses. It originates from the locus coeruleus and projects to various brain regions, including the prefrontal cortex and hippocampus.
- **Role in Learning Disabilities**:
    - **ADHD**: Dysregulation of norepinephrine in the prefrontal cortex can impact attention and executive functions. Medications targeting norepinephrine reuptake, such as atomoxetine, are used to manage ADHD symptoms.
    - **Dyslexia**: Variations in norepinephrine levels can influence reading processes by affecting attention and cognitive control.

Serotonergic System

- **Function**: The serotonergic system involves serotonin (5-HT), which regulates mood, anxiety, and cognitive functions. Serotonin pathways originate from the raphe nuclei and project to many brain regions, including the

cortex and limbic system.
- **Role in Learning Disabilities**:
    - **ADHD**: Serotonin dysregulation can contribute to mood instability and impulsivity. Some ADHD treatments, such as selective serotonin reuptake inhibitors (SSRIs), target serotonin levels to manage symptoms.
    - **Dyslexia**: Serotonin has been implicated in mood and anxiety disorders that can co-occur with dyslexia, potentially impacting learning and academic performance.

Glutamatergic System

- **Function**: The glutamatergic system involves glutamate (Glu), the primary excitatory neurotransmitter in the brain. Glutamate is crucial for synaptic plasticity, learning, and memory. It acts on various receptors, including NMDA, AMPA, and kainate receptors.
- **Role in Learning Disabilities**:
    - **Dyslexia**: Alterations in glutamate signaling can affect synaptic plasticity and neural connectivity, influencing reading and language processing abilities.
    - **ADHD**: Glutamate system dysregulation can impact cognitive control and attention by affecting synaptic transmission and plasticity in the prefrontal cortex.

GABAergic System

- **Function**: The GABAergic system involves gamma-aminobutyric acid (GABA), the primary inhibitory neurotransmitter in the brain. GABAergic signaling regulates neuronal excitability and maintains balance between excitation and inhibition.
- **Role in Learning Disabilities**:
    - **ADHD**: Imbalances between excitatory and inhibitory neurotransmission can contribute to

impulsivity and hyperactivity. Dysregulation of GABAergic systems can affect attention and executive functions.

- **Dyslexia**: GABAergic dysfunction can influence neural circuits involved in reading and language processing by affecting inhibitory control and information processing.

2. Neurotransmitter Systems and Learning Disabilities

Dyslexia

- **Dopamine**: Abnormal dopamine signaling can affect cognitive control and processing speed, impacting reading abilities.
- **Glutamate**: Dysregulation in glutamate signaling can impair synaptic plasticity and connectivity in brain regions associated with reading.
- **GABA**: Altered GABAergic function can disrupt inhibitory control in neural circuits involved in language processing.

ADHD

- **Dopamine**: Abnormal dopamine function in the prefrontal cortex and striatum affects attention, impulse control, and executive functions.
- **Norepinephrine**: Dysregulation of norepinephrine can impact attention and stress responses, influencing ADHD symptoms.
- **Serotonin**: Serotonin imbalances can contribute to mood instability and impulsivity, affecting ADHD-related behaviors.

Dyscalculia

- **Glutamate**: Alterations in glutamate signaling can impact numerical processing and mathematical abilities by affecting synaptic plasticity in relevant brain areas.

- **Dopamine**: Dopamine system dysfunction may influence cognitive processes involved in mathematical reasoning and problem-solving.

3. Therapeutic Implications

Pharmacological Interventions

- **Medication**: Pharmacological treatments targeting neurotransmitter systems can help manage symptoms of learning disabilities. For example:
    - **ADHD**: Stimulant medications (e.g., methylphenidate, amphetamines) increase dopamine and norepinephrine levels to improve attention and impulse control.
    - **Dyslexia**: Medications targeting neurotransmitter imbalances may be explored to address cognitive control and processing speed.
- **Future Directions**: Ongoing research into neurotransmitter systems may lead to the development of new medications targeting specific neurotransmitter imbalances associated with learning disabilities.

Non-Pharmacological Interventions

- **Cognitive Training**: Cognitive training programs can enhance neurotransmitter function and improve cognitive skills related to learning disabilities. For example:
    - **Attention Training**: Programs targeting attention and executive functions can help manage ADHD symptoms and improve cognitive control.
- **Behavioral Interventions**: Behavioral therapies and educational strategies can support neurotransmitter balance and improve learning outcomes. For example:
    - **Multisensory Learning**: Approaches that integrate multiple sensory modalities can support cognitive processes and enhance

learning in individuals with dyslexia.

4. Future Research Directions

Neurotransmitter Imaging

- **Advancements**: Development of imaging techniques to visualize neurotransmitter systems in vivo will provide deeper insights into their role in learning disabilities. Techniques such as PET and MRI-based methods are being explored.

Genetic and Neurotransmitter Interactions

- **Research Focus**: Investigating how genetic variations impact neurotransmitter systems and contribute to learning disabilities will enhance understanding of their etiology and guide personalized interventions.

Personalized Medicine

- **Tailored Treatments**: Advances in understanding neurotransmitter systems will facilitate the development of personalized treatment approaches based on individual neurotransmitter profiles and genetic factors.

Conclusion

Neurotransmitter systems play a vital role in the development and manifestation of learning disabilities. Dysregulation of neurotransmitters such as dopamine, norepinephrine, serotonin, glutamate, and GABA can impact cognitive functions and contribute to various learning disabilities. Understanding these systems' roles provides valuable insights into the neurobiological mechanisms underlying learning disabilities and informs the development of targeted pharmacological and non-pharmacological interventions. Future research will continue to advance our understanding of neurotransmitter systems and their implications for personalized treatments and improved outcomes for individuals with learning disabilities.

Hormonal Influences and Endocrine Factors

Hormonal and endocrine factors play a significant role in shaping brain development, function, and, consequently, learning abilities. Hormones, which are chemical messengers secreted by endocrine glands, influence a range of physiological and psychological processes. Dysregulation of hormonal systems can impact cognitive functions and contribute to various learning disabilities. This section explores the effects of key hormones and endocrine factors on learning disabilities, including their mechanisms of action and implications for diagnosis and treatment.

1. Overview of Key Hormones and Endocrine Factors

Cortisol

- **Function**: Cortisol, a glucocorticoid hormone produced by the adrenal glands, is critical for regulating the body's response to stress. It affects various brain functions, including memory, attention, and emotional regulation.
- **Role in Learning Disabilities**:
  - **ADHD**: Elevated cortisol levels due to chronic stress or environmental factors can exacerbate symptoms of ADHD. High cortisol levels may impair cognitive functions related to attention and executive control.
  - **Dyslexia**: Chronic stress and high cortisol levels can negatively impact cognitive processes involved in reading and language development.
- **Mechanism**: Cortisol affects the hippocampus, a brain region crucial for learning and memory, by influencing synaptic plasticity and neuronal survival. Prolonged exposure to high cortisol levels can lead to hippocampal atrophy and cognitive impairments.

Thyroid Hormones

- **Function**: Thyroid hormones, including thyroxine (T4) and triiodothyronine (T3), are essential for normal brain development and function. They regulate metabolic processes, neuronal differentiation, and synaptic plasticity.
- **Role in Learning Disabilities**:
  - **Dyslexia**: Hypothyroidism during pregnancy or early childhood can affect brain development, leading to cognitive deficits and learning disabilities. Thyroid hormone levels influence language development and reading abilities.
  - **ADHD**: Thyroid dysfunction, including both hypo- and hyperthyroidism, can impact cognitive functions and contribute to ADHD symptoms by altering neurodevelopmental processes.
- **Mechanism**: Thyroid hormones regulate gene expression related to brain development and function. They affect the growth and maturation of neurons, synapse formation, and myelination.

Sex Hormones

- **Function**: Sex hormones, including estrogen and testosterone, influence brain development, cognitive function, and emotional regulation. These hormones vary across the lifespan and can affect learning processes differently in males and females.
- **Role in Learning Disabilities**:
  - **ADHD**: Variations in sex hormones can influence ADHD symptoms. For example, changes in estrogen levels during puberty can affect attention and impulsivity.
  - **Dyslexia**: Sex hormones may influence the prevalence and manifestation of dyslexia. Differences in estrogen and testosterone levels can impact reading abilities and cognitive processing.

- **Mechanism**: Sex hormones affect brain regions involved in cognitive functions and emotional regulation. Estrogen influences synaptic plasticity and neuronal growth, while testosterone affects cognitive functions and behavior.

Insulin and Glucose Regulation

- **Function**: Insulin, produced by the pancreas, regulates blood glucose levels and plays a role in brain function. Adequate glucose supply is essential for neuronal energy and cognitive processes.
- **Role in Learning Disabilities**:
    - **ADHD**: Impaired glucose metabolism and insulin resistance can affect cognitive functions, including attention and executive control. Disruptions in glucose regulation may exacerbate ADHD symptoms.
    - **Dyslexia**: Glucose metabolism and insulin levels may influence cognitive functions related to reading and language processing. Hypoglycemia or insulin resistance can impact learning abilities.
- **Mechanism**: Insulin and glucose levels affect brain energy metabolism, synaptic function, and cognitive processes. Disruptions in glucose regulation can impair cognitive functions and contribute to learning disabilities.

2. Mechanisms of Hormonal Influence on Learning Disabilities

Neurodevelopmental Impact

- **Brain Development**: Hormones influence brain development during critical periods, including prenatal and early postnatal stages. Dysregulation of hormonal systems can impact neuronal differentiation, synaptic formation, and brain connectivity.
- **Neuroplasticity**: Hormones affect synaptic plasticity

and neuronal remodeling, which are crucial for learning and memory. Imbalances in hormonal levels can disrupt these processes and contribute to learning disabilities.

Cognitive Functions

- **Attention and Executive Functions**: Hormones such as cortisol and thyroid hormones affect cognitive functions related to attention and executive control. Dysregulation can impair these functions, leading to learning difficulties.
- **Memory and Learning**: Hormones influence memory formation and learning processes by affecting brain regions such as the hippocampus and prefrontal cortex. Imbalances can impair cognitive performance and learning abilities.

Emotional and Behavioral Regulation

- **Stress and Anxiety**: Hormones involved in stress responses, such as cortisol, can impact emotional regulation and behavior. Chronic stress and elevated cortisol levels can exacerbate symptoms of learning disabilities and affect academic performance.
- **Mood Disorders**: Hormonal imbalances can contribute to mood disorders, which can impact learning and academic achievement. Addressing hormonal influences on mood and behavior is crucial for managing learning disabilities.

3. Diagnostic and Therapeutic Implications

Hormonal Assessment

- **Testing**: Evaluating hormonal levels through blood tests and other diagnostic tools can provide insights into potential endocrine factors contributing to learning disabilities. Testing for cortisol, thyroid hormones, sex hormones, and glucose levels can inform diagnosis and treatment.

- **Clinical Evaluation**: Comprehensive evaluation of hormonal influences should be part of the assessment for learning disabilities, particularly when there are signs of endocrine dysfunction or metabolic imbalances.

Treatment Approaches

- **Hormonal Therapy**: Addressing hormonal imbalances through hormone replacement or regulation therapy can improve cognitive functions and learning outcomes. For example:
  - **Thyroid Hormone Replacement**: Treating hypothyroidism with thyroid hormone replacement can mitigate cognitive deficits and support normal brain development.
  - **Stress Management**: Interventions to manage stress and regulate cortisol levels can improve cognitive functions and academic performance in individuals with learning disabilities.
- **Lifestyle and Dietary Interventions**: Managing diet and lifestyle factors, such as glucose regulation and stress reduction, can support hormonal balance and improve learning outcomes.

4. Future Research Directions

Understanding Hormonal Interactions

- **Complex Interactions**: Research into how different hormones interact and influence brain development and function will enhance understanding of their role in learning disabilities. Examining the interplay between cortisol, thyroid hormones, sex hormones, and other factors will provide a more comprehensive view.

Personalized Treatments

- **Tailored Approaches**: Advances in understanding hormonal influences will lead to more personalized treatment approaches for learning disabilities. Tailoring interventions based on individual hormonal profiles and needs will improve outcomes.

Preventive Strategies

- **Early Intervention**: Identifying and addressing hormonal imbalances early in development can prevent or mitigate the impact of learning disabilities. Implementing preventive strategies based on hormonal assessments will support healthy brain development and cognitive function.

Conclusion

Hormonal and endocrine factors play a significant role in the development and manifestation of learning disabilities. Hormones such as cortisol, thyroid hormones, sex hormones, and insulin influence brain development, cognitive functions, and emotional regulation. Dysregulation of these hormonal systems can impact learning abilities and contribute to various learning disabilities. Understanding the mechanisms through which hormones affect learning and behavior provides valuable insights for diagnosis and treatment. Future research will continue to enhance our knowledge of hormonal influences and lead to more effective and personalized approaches to managing learning disabilities.

Epigenetic Modifications and Learning Disabilities

Epigenetic modifications involve changes in gene expression that do not alter the DNA sequence but affect how genes are turned on or off. These modifications can influence brain development and cognitive functions, making them critical to understanding learning disabilities. This section delves into the nature of epigenetic modifications, their role in learning disabilities, and their implications for diagnosis and treatment.

1. Overview of Epigenetic Mechanisms

DNA Methylation

- **Function**: DNA methylation involves the addition of a

methyl group to the DNA molecule, typically at cytosine residues within CpG dinucleotides. This process can inhibit gene expression by preventing the binding of transcription factors and other regulatory proteins.

- **Role in Learning Disabilities**: Abnormal DNA methylation patterns can affect genes involved in brain development and cognitive functions. For example:
    - **ADHD**: Altered DNA methylation of genes associated with neurotransmitter systems, such as dopamine and norepinephrine receptors, can influence attention and impulse control.
    - **Dyslexia**: DNA methylation changes in genes related to language processing and reading can contribute to difficulties in these areas.
- **Mechanism**: Changes in DNA methylation can impact gene expression in neurons, affecting processes such as synaptic plasticity, neuronal differentiation, and cognitive development.

Histone Modifications

- **Function**: Histone modifications involve chemical changes to histone proteins around which DNA is wrapped. These modifications, including acetylation, methylation, and phosphorylation, affect chromatin structure and gene accessibility.
- **Role in Learning Disabilities**: Abnormal histone modifications can alter the expression of genes crucial for brain function. For example:
    - **Dyslexia**: Changes in histone acetylation can affect genes involved in neural development and language processing.
    - **ADHD**: Histone modifications influencing the expression of genes related to neurotransmitter systems can impact attention and executive functions.

- **Mechanism**: Histone modifications can influence chromatin structure, affecting the accessibility of genes involved in cognitive functions and brain development.

Non-Coding RNAs

- **Function**: Non-coding RNAs, such as microRNAs (miRNAs) and long non-coding RNAs (lncRNAs), regulate gene expression by binding to mRNA molecules and influencing their stability or translation.
- **Role in Learning Disabilities**: Non-coding RNAs can affect genes involved in neural development and cognitive functions. For example:
    - **ADHD**: Dysregulation of miRNAs that target genes involved in neurotransmitter systems can impact attention and behavior.
    - **Dyslexia**: Alterations in lncRNAs related to language processing and reading abilities can contribute to dyslexia.
- **Mechanism**: Non-coding RNAs modulate gene expression and neuronal function by affecting the stability and translation of mRNAs involved in brain development and cognitive processes.

2. Epigenetic Modifications and Learning Disabilities

Dyslexia

- **Gene Expression**: Epigenetic modifications can affect genes involved in reading and language processing. For example:
    - **DNA Methylation**: Changes in DNA methylation of genes such as DYX1C1, KIAA0319, and ROBO1, which are associated with dyslexia, can impact their expression and contribute to reading difficulties.
    - **Histone Modifications**: Alterations in histone acetylation or methylation can influence the expression of genes crucial for neural development and language skills.

- **Neurodevelopmental Impact**: Epigenetic changes can affect neuronal differentiation, synaptic plasticity, and connectivity, impacting cognitive processes related to reading and language.

ADHD

- **Neurotransmitter Systems**: Epigenetic modifications can influence the expression of genes related to neurotransmitter systems, such as dopamine and norepinephrine receptors. For example:
    - **DNA Methylation**: Changes in DNA methylation of genes like DRD4 and DAT1 can affect neurotransmitter function and contribute to ADHD symptoms.
    - **Non-Coding RNAs**: Dysregulation of miRNAs targeting neurotransmitter-related genes can impact attention, impulse control, and executive functions.
- **Behavioral and Cognitive Impact**: Epigenetic changes can affect brain regions involved in attention and executive functions, leading to symptoms of ADHD.

Dyscalculia

- **Mathematical Processing**: Epigenetic modifications can influence genes involved in numerical cognition and mathematical processing. For example:
    - **Histone Modifications**: Changes in histone modifications affecting genes related to mathematical abilities can contribute to dyscalculia.
    - **Non-Coding RNAs**: Alterations in non-coding RNAs involved in numerical cognition can impact mathematical processing and problem-solving skills.
- **Neurodevelopmental Impact**: Epigenetic changes can affect neural circuits involved in numerical cognition and mathematical abilities, contributing to difficulties

in these areas.

3. Environmental Influences on Epigenetic Modifications

Prenatal and Early Life Factors

- **Nutrition and Toxins**: Prenatal exposure to factors such as poor nutrition, toxins, or stress can lead to epigenetic modifications that impact brain development and learning abilities. For example:
    - **Nutrition**: Maternal nutrition can affect DNA methylation patterns and gene expression related to brain development.
    - **Toxins**: Exposure to environmental toxins during pregnancy can lead to epigenetic changes that impact cognitive development.
- **Mechanism**: Environmental factors can influence epigenetic modifications, affecting gene expression and contributing to learning disabilities.

Educational and Social Environments

- **Learning Experiences**: Early educational experiences and social interactions can impact epigenetic modifications related to cognitive functions. For example:
    - **Stress and Trauma**: Chronic stress and trauma can lead to epigenetic changes that affect cognitive development and learning abilities.
    - **Enriched Environments**: Positive educational experiences and supportive environments can modulate epigenetic modifications and enhance learning outcomes.
- **Mechanism**: Environmental influences can affect gene expression through epigenetic modifications, impacting brain development and cognitive functions.

4. Diagnostic and Therapeutic Implications

Epigenetic Assessment

- **Biomarkers**: Identifying epigenetic biomarkers

associated with learning disabilities can provide insights into their underlying mechanisms and inform diagnosis. For example:
  - **DNA Methylation Patterns**: Analyzing DNA methylation patterns of genes related to learning disabilities can help identify individuals at risk and understand their condition.
- **Clinical Evaluation**: Incorporating epigenetic assessments into clinical evaluations can enhance the understanding of learning disabilities and guide treatment strategies.

Therapeutic Approaches

- **Epigenetic Therapies**: Developing therapies that target epigenetic modifications can offer new treatment options for learning disabilities. For example:
  - **Pharmacological Interventions**: Drugs that modify DNA methylation or histone acetylation can potentially be used to address epigenetic dysregulation in learning disabilities.
  - **Lifestyle Interventions**: Nutritional and lifestyle interventions that influence epigenetic modifications can support cognitive development and improve learning outcomes.

Preventive Strategies

- **Early Intervention**: Identifying and addressing environmental factors that impact epigenetic modifications can prevent or mitigate learning disabilities. For example:
  - **Prenatal Care**: Ensuring optimal prenatal care and reducing exposure to toxins can support healthy epigenetic profiles and brain development.
  - **Educational Support**: Providing supportive educational environments can enhance cognitive development and modulate

epigenetic modifications.

5. Future Research Directions

Epigenetic Mechanisms

- **Understanding Complex Interactions**: Further research into the complex interactions between genetic, epigenetic, and environmental factors will enhance understanding of learning disabilities. Examining how different epigenetic modifications interact with genetic and environmental influences will provide a more comprehensive view.

Translational Research

- **Clinical Applications**: Translating findings from epigenetic research into clinical practice will lead to new diagnostic tools and therapeutic strategies for learning disabilities. Developing epigenetic-based interventions will improve treatment options and outcomes.

Personalized Medicine

- **Tailored Approaches**: Advances in epigenetics will facilitate personalized treatment approaches based on individual epigenetic profiles. Tailoring interventions to address specific epigenetic modifications will enhance the effectiveness of treatments for learning disabilities.

Conclusion

Epigenetic modifications play a crucial role in the development and manifestation of learning disabilities. Changes in DNA methylation, histone modifications, and non-coding RNAs can influence gene expression and impact cognitive functions. Understanding these epigenetic mechanisms provides valuable insights into the underlying causes of learning disabilities and informs the development of diagnostic and therapeutic strategies. Future research will continue to enhance our knowledge of epigenetic influences and lead to more effective and personalized approaches to managing learning disabilities.

CHAPTER 4: COGNITIVE AND PSYCHOLOGICAL MECHANISMS

Cognitive Theories of Learning Disabilities

Cognitive theories of learning disabilities focus on understanding how cognitive processes such as perception, memory, and executive function contribute to difficulties in learning. These theories provide a framework for analyzing how deficits in cognitive processes can lead to specific learning disabilities, such as dyslexia, ADHD, and dyscalculia. This section explores key cognitive theories, their relevance to learning disabilities, and how they inform assessment and intervention strategies.

1. Overview of Cognitive Processes in Learning

Attention

- **Function**: Attention is a cognitive process that involves selectively focusing on specific information while ignoring irrelevant stimuli. It is critical for encoding, maintaining, and retrieving information.
- **Relevance to Learning Disabilities**: Deficits in attention can lead to difficulties in acquiring and processing new information. For instance:
    - **ADHD**: Individuals with ADHD often exhibit impairments in sustained and selective attention, which affect their ability to focus on

tasks and follow instructions.
- **Dyslexia**: Attention deficits can impact reading fluency and comprehension by making it difficult to maintain focus on written text.

Memory

- **Function**: Memory involves encoding, storing, and retrieving information. It encompasses different types, including working memory, short-term memory, and long-term memory.
- **Relevance to Learning Disabilities**: Impairments in memory can hinder learning by affecting the ability to retain and recall information. For example:
    - **Dyslexia**: Difficulties in phonological working memory can affect the ability to decode and remember words, impacting reading abilities.
    - **ADHD**: Deficits in working memory can lead to problems with organizing and retaining information, affecting task completion and academic performance.

Executive Functions

- **Function**: Executive functions are high-level cognitive processes that include planning, organization, problem-solving, and cognitive flexibility. These functions enable individuals to manage and regulate their thoughts and actions.
- **Relevance to Learning Disabilities**: Impairments in executive functions can affect a wide range of learning activities, including task initiation, organization, and self-monitoring. For example:
    - **ADHD**: Executive function deficits, such as poor planning and impulse control, are central to the challenges faced by individuals with ADHD.
    - **Dyscalculia**: Executive function difficulties can impact mathematical problem-solving and organization of numerical information.

2. Cognitive Theories of Specific Learning Disabilities

Dyslexia

- **Phonological Processing Theory**
    - **Concept**: This theory posits that difficulties with phonological processing—such as recognizing and manipulating sounds in spoken language—underlie dyslexia. Phonological awareness is crucial for decoding written words.
    - **Evidence**: Research shows that individuals with dyslexia often have impaired phonological processing skills, which affects their ability to read and spell.
- **Double-Deficit Hypothesis**
    - **Concept**: This hypothesis suggests that dyslexia may result from both a phonological deficit and a naming speed deficit. The combined effect of these two deficits contributes to reading difficulties.
    - **Evidence**: Studies have shown that individuals with dyslexia often struggle with rapid naming tasks in addition to phonological processing.

ADHD

- **Inattentional Theory**
    - **Concept**: Inattentional theory suggests that ADHD is characterized by deficits in attention and the ability to sustain focus on tasks. This leads to difficulties with task completion and performance.
    - **Evidence**: Neuropsychological research indicates that individuals with ADHD exhibit reduced activation in brain areas associated with attention and executive control.
- **Executive Function Theory**
    - **Concept**: This theory proposes that ADHD is related to deficits in executive functions, including working memory, inhibition, and

cognitive flexibility. These impairments affect planning and organizational skills.
- **Evidence**: Neuroimaging studies have identified structural and functional abnormalities in brain regions responsible for executive functions in individuals with ADHD.

Dyscalculia

- **Number Sense Theory**
  - **Concept**: This theory posits that dyscalculia results from impairments in the innate number sense, or the ability to perceive and understand numerical quantities. Deficits in number sense can affect mathematical skills.
  - **Evidence**: Research indicates that individuals with dyscalculia have difficulty with basic numerical concepts and arithmetic operations, suggesting a core deficit in number sense.

- **Working Memory Theory**
  - **Concept**: This theory suggests that difficulties in working memory contribute to dyscalculia by impairing the ability to hold and manipulate numerical information during problem-solving.
  - **Evidence**: Studies have shown that individuals with dyscalculia often have deficits in working memory related to numerical and arithmetic processing.

3. Implications for Assessment and Intervention

Assessment

- **Cognitive Testing**: Assessing cognitive processes such as attention, memory, and executive functions can help identify specific deficits contributing to learning disabilities. For example:
  - **Attention**: Tests measuring sustained and selective attention can help diagnose ADHD and inform treatment strategies.

- **Memory**: Assessments of working memory and phonological memory can aid in diagnosing dyslexia and dyscalculia.
- **Functional Assessments**: Evaluating how cognitive deficits impact academic performance and daily functioning can provide a comprehensive understanding of the learning disability. Functional assessments can guide intervention planning and support.

Intervention

- **Targeted Interventions**: Cognitive theories inform targeted interventions aimed at addressing specific deficits. For example:
    - **Dyslexia**: Interventions may focus on improving phonological processing skills through phonics-based instruction and reading strategies.
    - **ADHD**: Interventions may include strategies to enhance attention and executive functions, such as behavioral therapy, organizational skills training, and medication.
    - **Dyscalculia**: Interventions may involve strategies to improve number sense and working memory, such as visual aids, practice with numerical concepts, and mathematical problem-solving techniques.
- **Educational Accommodations**: Tailoring educational accommodations to support cognitive weaknesses can improve learning outcomes. Examples include:
    - **Extended Time**: Providing additional time for tests and assignments to accommodate working memory and processing speed deficits.
    - **Assistive Technology**: Using tools such as text-to-speech software and organizational apps to support learning and task completion.

4. **Future Directions in Cognitive Theories of Learning**

Disabilities

Integration of Cognitive and Neurobiological Research

- **Cross-Disciplinary Approaches**: Combining cognitive theories with neurobiological research can enhance understanding of learning disabilities. Exploring how cognitive deficits relate to brain function and structure will provide a more comprehensive view.

Personalized Interventions

- **Tailored Approaches**: Advances in cognitive research will facilitate personalized interventions based on individual cognitive profiles. Tailoring interventions to specific cognitive strengths and weaknesses will improve effectiveness.

Longitudinal Studies

- **Developmental Perspectives**: Longitudinal studies examining how cognitive processes evolve over time in individuals with learning disabilities will provide insights into developmental trajectories and inform early intervention strategies.

Conclusion

Cognitive theories of learning disabilities offer valuable insights into the underlying cognitive processes that contribute to difficulties in learning. By understanding how deficits in attention, memory, and executive functions impact learning, educators and clinicians can develop targeted assessment and intervention strategies. Continued research into cognitive processes and their relationship to learning disabilities will enhance our ability to support individuals with learning challenges and improve educational outcomes.

Memory and Learning Processes

Memory is a cornerstone of learning, playing a critical role in how information is acquired, retained, and applied. Different types of memory contribute uniquely to learning processes, and impairments in these memory systems can lead to learning disabilities. In this section, we will explore the types of memory, the processes involved in memory formation and retrieval, and how these relate to learning.

1. Types of Memory and Their Functions in Learning

Sensory Memory

- **Function**: Sensory memory acts as the initial stage in the memory process, capturing fleeting impressions of sensory information from the environment. This memory is highly transient, lasting only a few milliseconds to a couple of seconds.
- **Role in Learning**: Sensory memory enables the brain to briefly hold onto sensory stimuli (e.g., sights, sounds) long enough for them to be transferred into short-term memory. For instance, when reading, sensory memory allows us to perceive letters and words before they are processed for meaning.

Short-Term Memory (STM) and Working Memory

- **Function**: Short-term memory temporarily holds information that is being processed. Working memory, a component of STM, actively manipulates and manages this information to perform cognitive tasks.
- **Role in Learning**: Working memory is crucial for tasks that require holding and manipulating information, such as solving math problems, following directions, or understanding language. It allows for the integration of new information with previously learned material, supporting comprehension and problem-solving.

Long-Term Memory (LTM)

- **Function**: Long-term memory is responsible for the storage of information over extended periods, ranging from hours to a lifetime. It is divided into explicit (declarative) memory, which includes episodic (personal experiences) and semantic (factual knowledge) memory, and implicit (non-declarative) memory, which includes procedural memory (skills and tasks).

- **Role in Learning**: Long-term memory is essential for the retention of knowledge and skills. Explicit memory allows for the recall of facts and events, which is fundamental in education, while implicit memory supports the automaticity of learned skills, such as reading or riding a bike.

2. Memory Processes in Learning

Encoding

- **Definition**: Encoding is the process by which sensory input is transformed into a form that can be stored in memory. Effective encoding involves attention, elaboration, and the use of mnemonic strategies.
- **Impact on Learning**: The quality of encoding determines how well information is stored and later retrieved. For example, students who engage in deep processing, such as relating new information to what they already know, are more likely to remember it. Inadequate encoding, often seen in learning disabilities, can result in poor retention and retrieval.

Storage

- **Definition**: Storage refers to the maintenance of encoded information over time. It involves the consolidation of memories, which can be influenced by factors such as sleep, repetition, and emotional significance.
- **Impact on Learning**: Effective storage is necessary for the long-term retention of information. Problems in storage, such as those found in some learning

disabilities, can lead to difficulties in recalling information, even if it was initially encoded correctly.

Retrieval

- **Definition**: Retrieval is the process of accessing stored information when it is needed. Retrieval can be either recall (bringing information to mind without cues) or recognition (identifying information when presented with cues).
- **Impact on Learning**: Successful retrieval depends on how well the information was encoded and stored. Learning disabilities can manifest as difficulties in retrieving information, leading to challenges in recalling facts during tests or applying knowledge in new situations.

3. Memory Impairments and Learning Disabilities

Dyslexia and Memory Deficits

- **Phonological Working Memory**: Dyslexia is often associated with deficits in phonological working memory, which is critical for holding and manipulating sound-based information. This can lead to difficulties in decoding and recognizing words, affecting reading fluency and comprehension.
- **Long-Term Memory and Retrieval**: Dyslexic individuals may also struggle with the retrieval of phonological information from long-term memory, which can impair their ability to recall spelling patterns or word meanings.

ADHD and Memory Challenges

- **Working Memory Deficits**: ADHD is frequently linked to deficits in working memory, particularly in the ability to hold and manipulate information over short periods. This can result in difficulties with following multi-step instructions, organizing tasks, and retaining information during problem-solving.

- **Encoding and Retrieval**: Individuals with ADHD may also experience challenges with encoding information due to inattentiveness, leading to poor storage and retrieval of information, which impacts learning and academic performance.

Dyscalculia and Memory Issues

- **Numerical Working Memory**: Dyscalculia is often related to deficits in working memory specific to numerical information. This affects the ability to hold and manipulate numbers in mind, leading to difficulties in arithmetic and problem-solving.
- **Procedural Memory**: Dyscalculia may also involve impairments in procedural memory, making it difficult to automate mathematical processes, such as multiplication tables or calculation methods.

4. Enhancing Memory in Learning

Mnemonic Strategies

- **Definition**: Mnemonics are memory aids that enhance encoding, storage, and retrieval. Techniques include acronyms, visualization, and chunking.
- **Application in Learning**: Educators can teach mnemonic strategies to help students encode and retrieve information more effectively. For example, using acronyms to remember lists or visual imagery to associate concepts can improve recall.

Repetition and Spaced Learning

- **Definition**: Repetition involves practicing information multiple times, while spaced learning distributes learning sessions over time, rather than cramming.
- **Application in Learning**: These techniques enhance memory consolidation, making it easier to store

information in long-term memory. Spaced repetition, in particular, has been shown to significantly improve retention.

Cognitive Load Management

- **Definition**: Cognitive load refers to the amount of working memory used during learning. Managing cognitive load involves breaking information into smaller, more manageable chunks.
- **Application in Learning**: Reducing cognitive load through techniques such as scaffolding and segmenting content can help students with memory deficits process and retain information more effectively.

Multisensory Learning

- **Definition**: Multisensory learning involves using multiple senses (visual, auditory, kinesthetic) to enhance memory encoding and retrieval.
- **Application in Learning**: This approach is particularly beneficial for students with learning disabilities, as it provides multiple pathways for memory retrieval. For instance, using both visual aids and hands-on activities can reinforce memory and understanding.

5. Future Directions in Memory Research and Learning Disabilities

Neurobiological Research

- **Advances**: Ongoing research into the neurobiological underpinnings of memory can provide deeper insights into how memory processes are affected in learning disabilities. For instance, understanding how different brain regions contribute to memory storage and retrieval can inform targeted interventions.

Personalized Learning Interventions

- **Customized Strategies**: Future developments may allow

for more personalized learning interventions that take into account individual memory strengths and weaknesses. Tailoring educational approaches based on a student's specific memory profile could enhance learning outcomes.

Technology and Memory Enhancement

- **Digital Tools**: Emerging technologies, such as cognitive training apps and adaptive learning platforms, can be used to strengthen memory processes. These tools can provide customized exercises that target specific memory deficits, supporting learners with disabilities in improving their memory functions.

Conclusion

Memory plays an integral role in the learning process, and understanding the different types and processes of memory is essential for addressing learning disabilities. By recognizing how memory deficits contribute to learning challenges, educators and clinicians can develop targeted interventions that enhance memory function and, consequently, learning outcomes. As research in memory and learning continues to evolve, there will be greater opportunities to support individuals with learning disabilities through personalized and evidence-based strategies.

Executive Functioning and Self-Regulation

Executive functioning and self-regulation are critical components of cognitive processing that significantly influence learning and behavior. These higher-order cognitive processes enable individuals to manage their thoughts, emotions, and actions to achieve goals and adapt to changing situations. In this section, we will explore the nature of executive functions, their role in self-regulation, how deficits in these areas can lead to learning disabilities, and strategies for enhancing executive functioning in educational settings.

1. Overview of Executive Functions

Definition and Components

- **Definition**: Executive functions are a set of cognitive processes that govern goal-directed behavior and enable individuals to plan, organize, make decisions, solve problems, and control impulses. These functions are often described as the "management system" of the brain.
- **Components**: The main components of executive functioning include:
    - **Inhibitory Control**: The ability to suppress impulsive responses and resist distractions.
    - **Working Memory**: The capacity to hold and manipulate information over short periods.
    - **Cognitive Flexibility**: The ability to shift attention between tasks or adapt to new situations.
    - **Planning and Organization**: The ability to set goals, develop strategies, and manage time and resources effectively.
    - **Self-Monitoring**: The ability to assess one's own performance and behavior in real-time and make adjustments as needed.

Neuroanatomical Basis

- **Prefrontal Cortex**: The prefrontal cortex, located at the front of the brain, is primarily responsible for executive functions. It is involved in decision-making, impulse control, and goal-directed behavior.
- **Anterior Cingulate Cortex**: This region is associated with error detection, conflict monitoring, and decision-making under uncertainty.
- **Basal Ganglia**: The basal ganglia play a role in motor control and habit formation, as well as in cognitive functions related to action selection and initiation.
- **Connections with Other Brain Regions**: Executive

functions rely on extensive networks connecting the prefrontal cortex with other brain areas, such as the limbic system (involved in emotions) and the parietal cortex (involved in spatial reasoning).

2. Role of Executive Functioning in Learning

Inhibitory Control and Attention

- **Function**: Inhibitory control helps individuals focus on relevant information while ignoring distractions, which is crucial for effective learning.
- **Impact on Learning**: Deficits in inhibitory control can lead to challenges such as difficulty staying on task, impulsive behavior, and trouble following instructions. For example, students with ADHD often struggle with inhibiting distractions, leading to poor academic performance.

Working Memory in Learning

- **Function**: Working memory is essential for temporarily holding information needed for complex cognitive tasks, such as problem-solving, comprehension, and reasoning.
- **Impact on Learning**: Impairments in working memory can hinder a student's ability to follow multi-step instructions, perform mental calculations, and retain information across lessons. This is particularly evident in learning disabilities like dyslexia and dyscalculia.

Cognitive Flexibility and Problem-Solving

- **Function**: Cognitive flexibility allows individuals to switch between different tasks, adapt to new rules, and consider multiple aspects of a problem simultaneously.
- **Impact on Learning**: Students with poor cognitive flexibility may struggle with transitioning between subjects, adapting to new learning environments, or

approaching problems from different angles. This rigidity can result in difficulties with subjects that require creative thinking or abstract reasoning, such as mathematics or writing.

Planning, Organization, and Goal Setting

- **Function**: Planning and organization involve setting goals, creating strategies to achieve them, and managing time and resources effectively.
- **Impact on Learning**: Students who have difficulties in planning and organization may find it challenging to complete assignments on time, break down tasks into manageable steps, or prioritize activities. This can lead to procrastination, missed deadlines, and academic underachievement.

Self-Monitoring and Self-Regulation

- **Function**: Self-monitoring allows students to evaluate their own performance and behavior and make adjustments as necessary. Self-regulation encompasses the ability to manage one's emotions, behavior, and cognitive processes to achieve long-term goals.
- **Impact on Learning**: Poor self-monitoring can result in students being unaware of their mistakes or learning needs, which hinders academic progress. Deficits in self-regulation can lead to emotional outbursts, difficulty managing stress, and challenges in maintaining focus during tasks.

3. Executive Functioning Deficits and Learning Disabilities

ADHD and Executive Dysfunction

- **Inhibitory Control and Impulsivity**: ADHD is characterized by significant deficits in inhibitory control, leading to impulsive behavior and difficulty sustaining attention. This can result in challenges in classroom settings, where students must remain focused and attentive for extended periods.

- **Working Memory Deficits**: Students with ADHD often struggle with working memory tasks, making it difficult to retain and manipulate information, follow multi-step instructions, and organize their thoughts.

Dyslexia and Executive Functions

- **Working Memory and Reading Comprehension**: Dyslexia is associated with working memory deficits, which can impact a student's ability to hold phonological information while decoding words, leading to difficulties with reading fluency and comprehension.
- **Cognitive Flexibility in Language Processing**: Students with dyslexia may also exhibit reduced cognitive flexibility, which can affect their ability to switch between different linguistic tasks, such as decoding unfamiliar words or understanding complex sentences.

Dyscalculia and Executive Functioning

- **Planning and Problem-Solving in Mathematics**: Dyscalculia often involves difficulties with executive functions related to planning and organizing numerical information, leading to challenges in solving math problems and understanding mathematical concepts.
- **Working Memory in Arithmetic**: Working memory deficits in dyscalculia can affect a student's ability to hold and manipulate numbers in their mind, making it difficult to perform calculations or remember mathematical procedures.

4. Enhancing Executive Functioning in Educational Settings

Teaching Strategies

- **Explicit Instruction in Executive Skills**: Teachers can explicitly teach executive functioning skills, such as planning, organization, and self-monitoring. This might involve modeling these skills, providing step-by-step instructions, and using visual aids to support learning.

- **Scaffolding and Support**: Providing scaffolding can help students gradually develop executive functioning skills. This might include breaking tasks into smaller, more manageable steps, providing regular feedback, and gradually increasing the complexity of tasks as students build their abilities.

Classroom Accommodations

- **Structured Environments**: Creating a structured classroom environment with clear routines and expectations can help students with executive functioning deficits manage their behavior and stay on task.
- **Use of Organizational Tools**: Tools such as planners, checklists, and graphic organizers can assist students in managing their time, organizing their work, and setting goals. For example, a daily planner can help students keep track of assignments and deadlines, while a graphic organizer can aid in breaking down complex tasks.

Interventions and Support Programs

- **Cognitive Behavioral Therapy (CBT)**: CBT can be effective in helping students develop better self-regulation and executive functioning skills by teaching them how to manage their thoughts and emotions and how to approach problems systematically.
- **Executive Function Coaching**: Some schools and educational programs offer executive function coaching, where students work one-on-one with a coach to develop strategies for improving their planning, organization, time management, and study skills.

Technology-Assisted Interventions

- **Digital Tools for Organization**: There are various apps and digital tools designed to help students with executive functioning deficits. These can include task management apps, reminders, and time-tracking tools that help students manage their schedules and tasks more effectively.
- **Interactive Software for Cognitive Training**: Some software programs are designed to enhance executive functions through targeted cognitive training exercises. These programs can improve working memory, attention, and cognitive flexibility through repetitive practice and feedback.

5. Future Directions in Executive Function Research and Education

Personalized Learning Approaches

- **Tailoring Interventions**: As our understanding of executive functions in learning disabilities grows, there is potential for more personalized interventions that are tailored to the specific executive functioning profiles of individual students. This might involve custom-designed educational plans that focus on the unique strengths and weaknesses of each student.

Neurofeedback and Brain Stimulation

- **Emerging Technologies**: Neurofeedback and non-invasive brain stimulation techniques, such as transcranial magnetic stimulation (TMS), are being explored as potential interventions for improving executive functions. These technologies aim to enhance brain activity in regions associated with executive control, potentially offering new avenues for supporting students with executive functioning deficits.

Longitudinal Studies on Executive Functioning Development

- **Understanding Developmental Trajectories**:

Longitudinal research tracking the development of executive functions from early childhood through adolescence and into adulthood will provide deeper insights into how these skills evolve over time and how early interventions can support long-term academic and life success.

Conclusion

Executive functioning and self-regulation are essential for successful learning and adaptive behavior. Deficits in these areas can lead to significant challenges in educational settings, particularly for students with learning disabilities such as ADHD, dyslexia, and dyscalculia. By understanding the role of executive functions in learning and implementing strategies to support these skills, educators and clinicians can help students overcome obstacles and achieve their academic potential. As research continues to advance, new interventions and technologies hold promise for further enhancing executive functioning and self-regulation in students with learning disabilities.

Attention and Perception

Attention and perception are fundamental cognitive processes that play a critical role in learning. They are the mechanisms by which we filter, focus on, and interpret sensory information, ultimately influencing how we interact with our environment and acquire new knowledge. Deficits in attention and perception can significantly impact learning abilities, often contributing to or exacerbating learning disabilities. This section explores the intricacies of attention and perception, their neurobiological underpinnings, their role in learning, and how impairments in these processes can lead to challenges in academic and everyday contexts.

1. Understanding Attention

Definition and Types of Attention

- **Definition**: Attention is the cognitive process

of selectively concentrating on a specific aspect of information while ignoring other perceivable information. It is crucial for managing sensory input and allocating cognitive resources effectively.

- **Types of Attention**:
    - **Sustained Attention**: The ability to maintain focus on a task or stimulus over a prolonged period. This is essential for tasks that require continuous concentration, such as reading or listening to a lecture.
    - **Selective Attention**: The ability to focus on a specific stimulus while ignoring distractions. This is critical in environments with competing stimuli, such as a noisy classroom.
    - **Divided Attention**: The ability to process multiple stimuli or tasks simultaneously. This is often necessary for tasks like taking notes while listening to a lecture.
    - **Alternating Attention**: The capacity to switch focus between different tasks or stimuli. This is important in dynamic situations that require shifting attention, such as in problem-solving or during complex tasks.

Neuroanatomical Basis of Attention

- **Frontal Lobe**: The prefrontal cortex, particularly the dorsolateral prefrontal cortex, is heavily involved in attentional control, including the regulation of sustained and selective attention.
- **Parietal Lobe**: The parietal cortex is associated with spatial attention and the integration of sensory information. It plays a key role in guiding attention to relevant stimuli in the environment.
- **Thalamus**: The thalamus acts as a relay station for sensory information and is crucial for filtering and directing attention to relevant stimuli.

- **Anterior Cingulate Cortex (ACC)**: The ACC is involved in error detection, conflict monitoring, and the allocation of attentional resources, particularly in challenging or novel situations.

2. Understanding Perception

Definition and Types of Perception

- **Definition**: Perception is the process by which the brain interprets and organizes sensory information to form meaningful experiences. It allows us to make sense of the world around us and respond appropriately to environmental stimuli.
- **Types of Perception**:
  - **Visual Perception**: The ability to interpret and make sense of visual stimuli, such as shapes, colors, and spatial relationships. This is essential for tasks like reading, writing, and navigating the environment.
  - **Auditory Perception**: The ability to process and interpret sounds, including speech and environmental noises. This is critical for language comprehension, communication, and auditory learning.
  - **Tactile Perception**: The ability to perceive and interpret information through touch, such as texture, temperature, and pressure. This is important for activities that involve manual manipulation, like writing or using tools.
  - **Spatial Perception**: The ability to understand the spatial relationships between objects, including their size, distance, and orientation. This is important for tasks like geometry, navigation, and organizing physical spaces.

Neuroanatomical Basis of Perception

- **Occipital Lobe**: The primary visual cortex, located in the occipital lobe, is responsible for processing visual information. It plays a critical role in interpreting visual stimuli and enabling visual perception.

- **Temporal Lobe**: The temporal lobe houses the primary auditory cortex, which processes auditory information. It is essential for understanding speech and other sounds.
- **Parietal Lobe**: The parietal cortex integrates sensory information from different modalities, contributing to spatial perception and body awareness.
- **Somatosensory Cortex**: Located in the parietal lobe, this area processes tactile information and is essential for tactile perception.

3. The Role of Attention and Perception in Learning

Attention as a Gateway to Learning

- **Focus and Information Processing**: Attention serves as a gateway to learning by filtering and prioritizing sensory information, allowing the brain to focus on relevant stimuli while ignoring irrelevant distractions. This selective focus is crucial for effective information processing and memory formation.
- **Attention and Cognitive Load**: The ability to sustain attention directly impacts a student's capacity to handle cognitive load. For example, a student who can maintain attention during a complex lesson is more likely to comprehend and retain the material.

Perception and Interpretation of Learning Materials

- **Visual Perception and Reading**: Visual perception is fundamental to reading and writing. Students with visual perception difficulties may struggle with recognizing letters, following lines of text, or understanding visual representations in learning materials, such as graphs and diagrams.

- **Auditory Perception and Language Learning**: Auditory perception is key to language acquisition and comprehension. Students with auditory perception difficulties may have trouble distinguishing between similar sounds, understanding spoken instructions, or following conversations in noisy environments.
- **Spatial Perception and Mathematical Understanding**: Spatial perception is crucial for understanding mathematical concepts, such as geometry and measurement. Students with spatial perception deficits may find it challenging to visualize shapes, understand spatial relationships, or interpret diagrams and graphs.

4. Attention, Perception, and Learning Disabilities

ADHD and Attentional Deficits

- **Impact on Learning**: ADHD is characterized by impairments in various types of attention, particularly sustained and selective attention. These deficits can lead to difficulties in maintaining focus on tasks, following instructions, and completing assignments, which are common challenges in academic settings.
- **Inhibitory Control**: Students with ADHD often struggle with inhibitory control, which is the ability to suppress irrelevant stimuli and distractions. This can result in impulsive behavior and difficulty concentrating on tasks.

Dyslexia and Perceptual Challenges

- **Visual Perception**: Dyslexia is often associated with visual perception difficulties, such as trouble distinguishing letters and words that look similar (e.g., "b" and "d"). These perceptual challenges can make reading and writing particularly difficult.
- **Auditory Perception**: Dyslexia can also involve deficits in auditory perception, particularly in phonological

processing—the ability to recognize and manipulate sounds in language. This can impact a student's ability to decode words and develop reading fluency.

Sensory Processing Disorders

- **Sensory Modulation**: Some students with learning disabilities may also have sensory processing disorders, where they either over-respond or under-respond to sensory stimuli. For example, a student may become easily overwhelmed by background noise (auditory sensitivity) or may have difficulty processing tactile information, which can affect their ability to focus and learn.

- **Integration of Sensory Information**: Difficulties in integrating sensory information from different modalities can lead to challenges in tasks that require coordination of multiple senses, such as reading (which involves both visual and auditory processing) or writing (which involves visual and tactile processing).

5. Enhancing Attention and Perception in Learning

Strategies for Improving Attention

- **Mindfulness and Attention Training**: Mindfulness practices can help students improve their ability to sustain attention by teaching them to focus on the present moment and reduce distractions. Techniques such as deep breathing, meditation, and guided imagery can be incorporated into the classroom to help students enhance their attentional control.

- **Structured Learning Environments**: Creating a structured and predictable learning environment can support students with attentional difficulties. This might include minimizing distractions, providing clear and concise instructions, and using visual or auditory cues to guide students' focus.

Interventions for Perceptual Difficulties

- **Visual Perception Training**: Exercises that improve visual discrimination, such as matching shapes, tracing letters, or working with puzzles, can enhance visual perception skills. These activities can help students with dyslexia or other visual processing disorders develop stronger reading and writing abilities.

- **Auditory Perception Enhancement**: Auditory training programs that focus on phonological awareness, such as distinguishing sounds or practicing sound-letter correspondence, can support students with auditory perception difficulties. These interventions are particularly beneficial for students with dyslexia or language processing disorders.

- **Multisensory Learning Approaches**: Incorporating multisensory learning approaches, such as using tactile, visual, and auditory inputs simultaneously, can help reinforce learning for students with perceptual difficulties. For example, using manipulatives in math instruction or integrating movement with reading activities can enhance comprehension and retention.

Assistive Technology for Attention and Perception

- **Digital Tools for Focus and Attention**: Apps and software that provide timers, reminders, and task management support can help students with attentional difficulties stay organized and on task. These tools can break down tasks into smaller, manageable steps, making it easier for students to maintain focus.

- **Assistive Devices for Sensory Processing**: Devices such as noise-canceling headphones, sensory cushions, or fidget tools can help students manage sensory overload and improve their ability to focus in the classroom. These tools can be particularly beneficial for students with sensory processing disorders or ADHD.

6. Future Directions in Research on Attention, Perception, and Learning

Neurodevelopmental Research

- **Advances in Neuroimaging**: Ongoing neuroimaging research is providing deeper insights into the neural networks involved in attention and perception. Understanding the specific brain mechanisms that underlie these processes can lead to more targeted interventions for students with learning disabilities.
- **Early Identification and Intervention**: Research into early markers of attention and perception deficits could enable earlier identification of at-risk students, allowing for timely interventions that can mitigate the impact of these deficits on learning outcomes.

Personalized Learning and Adaptive Technologies

- **Adaptive Learning Systems**: Emerging technologies are enabling the development of adaptive learning systems that can adjust to individual students' attentional and perceptual needs. These systems use data on student performance to tailor instructional materials and provide personalized support, enhancing learning outcomes.
- **Virtual Reality (VR) for Perceptual Training**: VR technology is being explored as a tool for perceptual training, offering immersive environments where students can practice visual, auditory, and spatial perception skills in a controlled and engaging manner.

Conclusion

Attention and perception are foundational to the learning process, influencing how students engage with and interpret educational materials. Deficits in these areas can lead to significant challenges, particularly for students with learning disabilities. By understanding the underlying mechanisms of attention and perception and implementing targeted interventions and strategies, educators and clinicians can better support students in overcoming these challenges and achieving their academic potential. Future research and technological advances hold promise for further enhancing our ability to address attentional and perceptual difficulties in educational settings.

Emotional and Behavioral Correlates

The emotional and behavioral aspects of learning disabilities are often as critical as the cognitive challenges themselves. Emotional well-being and behavioral regulation are closely linked to academic success and social functioning. When learning disabilities are present, they frequently give rise to a range of emotional and behavioral difficulties that can complicate the educational experience and overall quality of life for affected individuals. This section explores the emotional and behavioral correlates of learning disabilities, examining the ways in which these conditions influence emotional health, behavior, and interpersonal relationships. Additionally, it discusses the importance of early intervention, strategies for support, and the implications for educators, parents, and clinicians.

1. Emotional Correlates of Learning Disabilities

Common Emotional Responses

- **Frustration and Anxiety**: Learning disabilities often lead to repeated academic failures and challenges, which can foster feelings of frustration and anxiety. Children and adults with learning disabilities may become anxious about their performance, fearing embarrassment or failure, which can further impede their ability to learn.
- **Low Self-Esteem**: Persistent academic struggles can erode self-esteem. Individuals with learning disabilities frequently compare themselves to their peers, leading to feelings of inadequacy and a diminished sense of self-

worth. This is particularly common when their efforts do not result in success, despite hard work.

- **Depression**: Chronic feelings of failure and low self-esteem can contribute to the development of depression. Adolescents and adults with learning disabilities are particularly vulnerable to depressive symptoms, which may manifest as sadness, hopelessness, withdrawal from social activities, and a lack of motivation.

- **Anger and Resentment**: When learning disabilities are not properly understood or accommodated, individuals may feel angry or resentful toward their educational environment, teachers, or even peers. This anger can stem from a sense of being unfairly treated or misunderstood.

Neurobiological Links Between Emotions and Learning Disabilities

- **Amygdala and Emotional Regulation**: The amygdala, a key brain structure involved in processing emotions, is often implicated in the emotional challenges associated with learning disabilities. Dysregulation in this area can lead to heightened emotional responses, such as anxiety or anger, which can exacerbate learning difficulties.

- **Prefrontal Cortex and Emotional Control**: The prefrontal cortex, responsible for higher-order cognitive functions like decision-making and emotional regulation, may not function optimally in individuals with learning disabilities. This can make it difficult for them to manage emotions effectively, leading to impulsive behaviors and difficulty coping with stress.

- **Cortisol and Stress Response**: Chronic stress associated with learning disabilities can lead to dysregulation of the hypothalamic-pituitary-adrenal (HPA) axis, resulting in elevated levels of cortisol, the body's stress hormone. High cortisol levels over time can impair cognitive function and exacerbate anxiety and depression.

2. Behavioral Correlates of Learning Disabilities

Disruptive Behaviors and ADHD

- **Inattention and Hyperactivity**: Attention-Deficit/Hyperactivity Disorder (ADHD) frequently co-occurs with learning disabilities. ADHD is characterized by difficulties with attention, impulsivity, and hyperactivity. These behaviors can be disruptive in educational settings, leading to challenges in completing tasks, following instructions, and maintaining focus during lessons.

- **Oppositional Defiant Disorder (ODD)**: Some children with learning disabilities may exhibit oppositional or defiant behaviors, often as a response to the frustration and stress of struggling academically. ODD is marked by patterns of angry, irritable moods, argumentative behavior, and vindictiveness toward authority figures.

- **Aggression and Conduct Problems**: In some cases, particularly when emotional needs are unmet or learning disabilities are not properly addressed, individuals may develop more serious behavioral issues, such as aggression or conduct disorders. These behaviors can include physical aggression, property destruction, and deceitfulness.

Internalizing vs. Externalizing Behaviors

- **Internalizing Behaviors**: These are directed inward and include withdrawal, anxiety, depression, and somatic complaints. Children who internalize their difficulties may become socially withdrawn, excessively worry about their performance, or complain of physical symptoms like headaches or stomachaches without a clear medical cause.

- **Externalizing Behaviors**: These are directed outward and include hyperactivity, aggression, and disruptive behaviors. Externalizing behaviors are more visible in classroom settings and often lead to disciplinary action. They may manifest as frequent temper tantrums, defiance, or talking out of turn.

Social Skills Deficits

- **Peer Relationships**: Learning disabilities can affect the ability to form and maintain positive peer relationships. Children with learning disabilities may struggle with social cues, leading to misunderstandings, social rejection, or bullying. Poor social skills can further isolate these children, leading to feelings of loneliness and exacerbating emotional problems.
- **Social Communication**: Deficits in social communication are common in individuals with learning disabilities, particularly in those with conditions like autism spectrum disorder (ASD). These individuals may have difficulty understanding and responding appropriately in social interactions, which can lead to social withdrawal or conflict.

3. Impact on Academic Performance and Long-Term Outcomes

Academic Avoidance and School Refusal

- **Avoidance Behaviors**: Emotional and behavioral difficulties often lead to avoidance of academic tasks. This can manifest as procrastination, incomplete assignments, or feigned illness to avoid attending school. Over time, this avoidance can result in significant academic underachievement and a widening gap between the student and their peers.
- **School Refusal**: In severe cases, anxiety and depression may lead to school refusal, where the child refuses to attend school altogether. This can have profound

implications for their educational trajectory and future opportunities.

Long-Term Psychological and Social Outcomes

- **Chronic Stress and Mental Health**: The chronic stress associated with managing learning disabilities and associated emotional and behavioral challenges can have long-term effects on mental health. Adults who experienced unaddressed learning disabilities as children may be at higher risk for anxiety disorders, depression, and substance abuse.
- **Employment and Independence**: Behavioral and emotional issues that persist into adulthood can impact employability and independence. Individuals with unresolved learning disabilities may struggle with job performance, workplace relationships, and maintaining stable employment.

Family and Relationship Dynamics

- **Impact on Family Dynamics**: The emotional and behavioral challenges of a child with a learning disability can strain family relationships. Parents may experience stress, guilt, or frustration, while siblings might feel neglected or resentful. This can lead to tension and conflict within the family unit.
- **Romantic Relationships and Friendships**: In adulthood, emotional and behavioral difficulties related to learning disabilities can affect romantic relationships and friendships. Issues such as poor emotional regulation, low self-esteem, and social communication deficits can make it challenging to maintain healthy and fulfilling relationships.

4. Strategies for Supporting Emotional and Behavioral Health

Early Identification and Intervention

- **Screening and Assessment**: Early identification of

emotional and behavioral difficulties is crucial for effective intervention. Comprehensive assessments that evaluate both cognitive and emotional functioning can help in developing tailored intervention plans.

- **Behavioral Interventions**: Behavioral interventions, such as Cognitive Behavioral Therapy (CBT), can be effective in addressing emotional and behavioral difficulties. CBT helps individuals recognize and change negative thought patterns and behaviors, improving emotional regulation and reducing anxiety and depression.

Classroom and School-Based Strategies

- **Positive Behavioral Interventions and Supports (PBIS)**: PBIS is a proactive approach that aims to improve school climate and promote positive behavior. It involves setting clear expectations, teaching appropriate behaviors, and reinforcing positive behaviors through rewards and recognition.

- **Social-Emotional Learning (SEL) Programs**: SEL programs teach students skills like emotional regulation, empathy, and problem-solving. Integrating SEL into the curriculum can help students with learning disabilities develop better emotional and social skills, reducing the likelihood of behavioral issues.

- **Accommodations and Modifications**: Providing appropriate accommodations, such as extended time on tests, quiet workspaces, and breaks during tasks, can help reduce frustration and anxiety for students with learning disabilities. These accommodations should be tailored to the individual's specific needs.

Family and Community Support

- **Parental Involvement**: Active parental involvement in the child's education can make a significant difference in managing emotional and behavioral difficulties. Parents can work closely with teachers and clinicians to monitor progress, reinforce positive behaviors at home, and provide emotional support.

- **Community Resources**: Access to community resources, such as support groups, counseling services, and recreational programs, can provide additional support for individuals with learning disabilities and their families. These resources can help build a strong support network and reduce the sense of isolation.

Holistic Approaches

- **Mind-Body Interventions**: Techniques such as mindfulness, yoga, and relaxation exercises can help manage stress and improve emotional regulation. These practices can be integrated into daily routines at home or in the classroom to promote overall well-being.
- **Nutritional and Lifestyle Factors**: Attention to nutritional and lifestyle factors, such as a balanced diet, regular physical activity, and adequate sleep, can also support emotional and behavioral health. Proper nutrition and regular exercise have been shown to improve mood, reduce anxiety, and enhance cognitive function.

5. Future Directions in Research and Practice

Neuroscientific Research on Emotion and Behavior

- **Brain-Behavior Relationships**: Ongoing research into the brain-behavior relationships in learning disabilities is essential for developing more effective interventions. Understanding the neural correlates of emotional and behavioral difficulties can lead to targeted therapies that address the root causes of these challenges.
- **Advances in Emotional Regulation Interventions**: Developing and refining interventions that enhance

emotional regulation, such as biofeedback and neurofeedback, could provide new tools for managing the emotional aspects of learning disabilities.

Integrating Emotional and Behavioral Health in Education

- **Holistic Educational Models**: Future educational models may increasingly integrate emotional and behavioral health into the standard curriculum, recognizing the importance of addressing these aspects alongside academic learning. Schools could adopt a more holistic approach, focusing on the overall well-being of the student.

- **Technology and Emotional Support**: The use of technology, such as apps and online platforms, to support emotional and behavioral health is an emerging area. These tools can provide personalized emotional support and behavioral interventions, making them accessible to a broader range of students.

Conclusion

The emotional and behavioral correlates of learning disabilities are complex and multifaceted, impacting every aspect of an individual's life, from academic performance to social relationships and long-term mental health. Understanding these correlates is essential for providing effective support and interventions. By addressing emotional and behavioral challenges in tandem with cognitive difficulties, educators, clinicians, and families can help individuals with learning disabilities achieve their full potential and lead fulfilling lives.

CHAPTER 5: EDUCATIONAL STRATEGIES AND INTERVENTIONS

Evidence-Based Educational Interventions

Evidence-based educational interventions are critical in addressing the diverse needs of students with learning disabilities. These interventions are grounded in rigorous research and have been shown to be effective in improving academic outcomes, cognitive functioning, and social-emotional development for individuals with learning disabilities. This section delves into the various evidence-based approaches used in educational settings, exploring their theoretical underpinnings, implementation strategies, and the outcomes they aim to achieve.

1. Importance of Evidence-Based Practices

Definition and Criteria for Evidence-Based Interventions

- **Definition**: Evidence-based educational interventions are strategies, practices, and programs that have been scientifically tested and proven effective through rigorous research. These interventions are designed to address specific learning challenges and are tailored to the individual needs of students.
- **Criteria**: To be considered evidence-based, an intervention must meet several key criteria:
    - **Empirical Support**: The intervention must have

been tested in controlled studies with peer-reviewed results demonstrating its efficacy.
- **Replicability**: The intervention should produce consistent results across different settings and populations.
- **Fidelity of Implementation**: The intervention must be implemented as intended, with adherence to the prescribed methods and procedures.
- **Measured Outcomes**: There should be clear, measurable outcomes that demonstrate the effectiveness of the intervention in improving academic, cognitive, or social-emotional functioning.

The Role of Evidence-Based Interventions in Special Education

- **Addressing Learning Gaps**: Evidence-based interventions are crucial for closing the learning gaps that students with learning disabilities often face. These interventions provide targeted support that helps students overcome specific challenges, such as difficulties with reading, writing, math, or executive functioning.
- **Personalized Learning**: Evidence-based practices enable the customization of educational experiences to meet the unique needs of each student. By using interventions that are tailored to individual strengths and weaknesses, educators can provide more effective support.
- **Improving Long-Term Outcomes**: Students who receive evidence-based interventions are more likely to experience improved academic performance, better self-esteem, and enhanced social skills. These outcomes contribute to long-term success in school and beyond.

2. Types of Evidence-Based Educational Interventions

Direct Instruction

- **Overview**: Direct Instruction (DI) is a highly structured, teacher-led approach that focuses on clear, explicit teaching of specific skills. It involves systematic teaching procedures, with lessons that are broken down into small, manageable steps. DI is particularly effective for students with learning disabilities who benefit from repetition and practice.
- **Implementation**: DI requires careful planning and scripting of lessons, with a focus on providing immediate feedback and correction. Teachers deliver content directly and systematically, ensuring that students master each step before moving on to more complex material.
- **Outcomes**: Research has shown that DI can significantly improve reading, math, and language skills in students with learning disabilities. It is especially effective for those who struggle with foundational skills, such as phonemic awareness, decoding, and basic math operations.

Response to Intervention (RTI)

- **Overview**: RTI is a multi-tiered approach to early identification and support for students with learning disabilities. It integrates assessment and intervention within a tiered system to maximize student achievement and reduce behavior problems. RTI is designed to provide early, systematic assistance to children who are struggling academically.
- **Implementation**: RTI involves three tiers of intervention:
  - **Tier 1**: Universal interventions that are applied to all students in the general education classroom. These are preventive and proactive measures designed to promote overall academic success.

- **Tier 2**: Targeted interventions for students who do not respond to Tier 1 strategies. These small group interventions are more intensive and are designed to address specific skill deficits.
- **Tier 3**: Intensive, individualized interventions for students who show minimal response to Tier 2. These are often one-on-one interventions tailored to the student's unique needs.

- **Outcomes**: RTI has been shown to be effective in reducing the number of students referred for special education services by providing timely interventions. It also improves academic outcomes by ensuring that students receive the support they need before falling significantly behind.

Cognitive Behavioral Interventions (CBI)

- **Overview**: Cognitive Behavioral Interventions (CBI) integrate cognitive and behavioral strategies to address the learning and emotional needs of students with learning disabilities. These interventions focus on changing maladaptive thoughts and behaviors, improving self-regulation, and enhancing problem-solving skills.

- **Implementation**: CBI involves teaching students cognitive strategies to manage their thoughts and behaviors, such as self-monitoring, goal-setting, and using positive self-talk. Behavioral components may include reinforcement, modeling, and role-playing to practice new skills.

- **Outcomes**: CBI has been shown to be effective in improving academic performance, particularly in students with learning disabilities who also exhibit behavioral or emotional challenges. It can also reduce anxiety, increase motivation, and enhance overall academic engagement.

Multisensory Instruction

- **Overview**: Multisensory Instruction involves engaging multiple senses (visual, auditory, tactile, and kinesthetic) simultaneously to enhance learning. This approach is based on the understanding that students with learning disabilities often benefit from learning experiences that incorporate multiple sensory modalities.
- **Implementation**: Multisensory Instruction can be implemented in various subjects, but it is especially prevalent in reading instruction (e.g., the Orton-Gillingham approach). Techniques might include tracing letters in sand while saying the letter sound, using manipulatives for math problems, or incorporating movement into learning activities.
- **Outcomes**: Research supports the effectiveness of multisensory instruction in improving reading and math skills, particularly for students with dyslexia or other reading disabilities. It helps reinforce learning by providing multiple pathways for information to be encoded and retrieved.

Peer-Assisted Learning Strategies (PALS)

- **Overview**: Peer-Assisted Learning Strategies (PALS) involve pairing students to work together on academic tasks, with one student taking on the role of tutor and the other as the tutee. This approach leverages peer interactions to reinforce learning, provide immediate feedback, and enhance motivation.
- **Implementation**: In PALS, students are typically paired based on their skill levels, with more proficient students guiding their peers through tasks. The roles of tutor and tutee are rotated to ensure that both students benefit from the interaction. Structured activities and prompts guide the sessions, ensuring that they are focused and

productive.

- **Outcomes**: PALS has been shown to improve reading and math skills, as well as social skills, in students with learning disabilities. The collaborative nature of the intervention helps build confidence and fosters a sense of community within the classroom.

3. Implementing Evidence-Based Interventions in Educational Settings

Fidelity of Implementation

- **Training and Professional Development**: Effective implementation of evidence-based interventions requires thorough training and ongoing professional development for educators. Teachers must be well-versed in the specific techniques and strategies associated with each intervention to ensure they are delivered with fidelity.
- **Monitoring and Support**: Schools should establish systems for monitoring the implementation of interventions, providing feedback, and offering support to educators. This might include regular observations, coaching, and data-driven discussions about student progress.

Individualized Education Programs (IEPs) and 504 Plans

- **Customized Interventions**: Evidence-based interventions should be integrated into a student's Individualized Education Program (IEP) or 504 Plan, ensuring that the strategies are aligned with the student's specific needs and goals. These plans should include clear objectives, timelines, and criteria for measuring success.
- **Collaboration with Specialists**: Collaboration between general education teachers, special education teachers, and other specialists (e.g., speech-language

pathologists, occupational therapists) is essential for the effective implementation of evidence-based interventions. Teamwork ensures that interventions are comprehensive and address all aspects of the student's needs.

Challenges and Considerations

- **Resource Allocation**: Implementing evidence-based interventions can require significant resources, including time, materials, and personnel. Schools must carefully allocate resources to ensure that all students who need interventions receive them without overburdening staff or compromising the quality of instruction.
- **Cultural and Linguistic Responsiveness**: Interventions must be culturally and linguistically responsive to be effective for all students. This involves adapting materials and approaches to be relevant and accessible to students from diverse backgrounds, ensuring that interventions are inclusive and equitable.

4. Measuring the Effectiveness of Educational Interventions

Data-Driven Decision Making

- **Progress Monitoring**: Regular progress monitoring is essential for assessing the effectiveness of interventions. This involves collecting and analyzing data on student performance to determine whether the intervention is meeting its intended goals.
- **Adjusting Interventions**: Based on data collected through progress monitoring, educators may need to adjust interventions to better meet the student's needs. This could involve increasing the intensity of the intervention, changing the instructional approach, or adding additional supports.

Longitudinal Studies and Meta-Analyses

- **Research on Long-Term Outcomes**: Longitudinal studies that track students over time are valuable for understanding the long-term effectiveness of evidence-based interventions. These studies can reveal how early interventions impact academic achievement, social-emotional development, and life outcomes.
- **Meta-Analyses of Intervention Effectiveness**: Meta-analyses that aggregate findings from multiple studies provide a broader understanding of the effectiveness of various interventions. These analyses can identify which interventions are most effective for different types of learning disabilities and in different educational contexts.

5. Future Directions in Evidence-Based Educational Interventions

Integrating Technology in Interventions

- **Adaptive Learning Technologies**: The use of technology in educational interventions is expanding, with adaptive learning platforms offering personalized instruction that adjusts to the student's progress in real-time. These technologies can provide additional support and practice opportunities outside of traditional classroom settings.
- **Virtual and Augmented Reality**: Emerging technologies like virtual and augmented reality are being explored as tools for enhancing evidence-based interventions. These technologies can create immersive learning environments that engage students and provide new ways to practice skills.

Expanding Research on Understudied Interventions

- **Innovative Approaches**: There is a need for continued research into innovative interventions that have not yet been widely studied. This includes interventions that incorporate new pedagogical theories, cross-disciplinary approaches, or novel technologies.

- **Focus on Diverse Populations**: More research is needed to understand how evidence-based interventions can be adapted for students from diverse cultural, linguistic, and socioeconomic backgrounds. Ensuring that interventions are effective for all students is crucial for promoting equity in education.

Conclusion

Evidence-based educational interventions play a crucial role in supporting students with learning disabilities, providing them with the tools and strategies they need to succeed academically and socially. By focusing on interventions that are grounded in rigorous research, educators can deliver more effective instruction that addresses the unique challenges faced by these students. Continued research, professional development, and the integration of new technologies will further enhance the ability of schools to provide high-quality, evidence-based support for all learners.

Special Education Techniques and Technologies

Special education is a dynamic field that has evolved significantly over the years, integrating a wide range of techniques and technologies to better serve students with learning disabilities. These advancements are aimed at providing personalized support, enhancing learning experiences, and fostering independence. This section explores the various specialized techniques and emerging technologies that are transforming special education, highlighting their applications, effectiveness, and the future of special education.

1. Overview of Special Education Techniques

Individualized Education Programs (IEPs)

- **Purpose and Structure**: Individualized Education

Programs (IEPs) are the cornerstone of special education. An IEP is a legally binding document that outlines the specific educational goals, services, accommodations, and modifications required for a student with a disability. Each IEP is tailored to meet the unique needs of the student, ensuring that they receive appropriate support to achieve academic success.

- **Key Components**: An IEP includes several critical components, such as the student's current level of academic performance, measurable annual goals, specific special education and related services to be provided, and the methods for measuring progress. The IEP is developed collaboratively by a team that includes educators, parents, and specialists.

- **Implementation and Review**: The implementation of an IEP requires careful coordination among teachers, special educators, and support staff. Regular reviews and updates to the IEP ensure that it remains relevant and effective as the student's needs evolve.

Differentiated Instruction

- **Definition and Approach**: Differentiated instruction is a teaching approach that involves tailoring instruction to meet the diverse needs of students within a classroom. This technique is particularly beneficial in special education, where students often have varying abilities, learning styles, and interests.

- **Strategies**: Differentiated instruction can be implemented through various strategies, such as flexible grouping, tiered assignments, and choice boards. Teachers may modify content, process, product, or the learning environment based on individual student needs.

- **Benefits**: Differentiated instruction helps ensure that all students, including those with learning disabilities, have access to the curriculum at an appropriate level of challenge. This approach promotes engagement, reduces frustration, and supports the development of each student's strengths.

Universal Design for Learning (UDL)

- **Principles of UDL**: Universal Design for Learning (UDL) is a framework for designing educational environments that are accessible and effective for all students, regardless of their abilities or disabilities. UDL is based on three key principles: providing multiple means of representation (how information is presented), multiple means of action and expression (how students demonstrate their knowledge), and multiple means of engagement (how students are motivated to learn).

- **Application in Special Education**: UDL is particularly effective in special education because it anticipates and addresses the diverse needs of students from the outset. By incorporating flexibility into the curriculum, UDL reduces the need for retroactive accommodations and ensures that all students can participate fully in their education.

- **Outcomes**: Implementing UDL in special education settings can lead to improved academic performance, greater student engagement, and a more inclusive learning environment. It also empowers students with learning disabilities to take ownership of their learning by providing them with choices and opportunities to demonstrate their understanding in ways that work best for them.

Assistive Technology (AT)

- **Definition and Types**: Assistive Technology (AT) encompasses a wide range of devices, tools, and software that support the learning and daily functioning of students with disabilities. AT can include low-tech solutions, such as pencil grips and graphic organizers, as well as high-tech tools, like speech-to-text software, screen readers, and communication devices.

- **Implementation**: The selection of AT is based on the individual needs of the student and is often included in their IEP. Educators, therapists, and technology specialists work together to identify the most appropriate tools and provide training on their use.

- **Impact on Learning**: AT can significantly enhance the learning experiences of students with disabilities by providing them with tools that compensate for their challenges, promote independence, and facilitate access to the curriculum. For example, students with dysgraphia might use speech-to-text software to complete writing assignments, while those with visual impairments might use screen readers to access digital content.

2. Emerging Technologies in Special Education

Augmented Reality (AR) and Virtual Reality (VR)

- **Overview**: Augmented Reality (AR) and Virtual Reality (VR) are cutting-edge technologies that are beginning to make their mark in special education. AR overlays digital content onto the real world, while VR immerses users in a fully simulated environment. Both technologies offer interactive and engaging ways to enhance learning experiences for students with disabilities.

- **Applications in Special Education**: AR and VR can be used to create simulations that help students with learning disabilities practice social skills, explore real-world scenarios in a safe environment, or visualize complex concepts in subjects like science and mathematics. For example, VR can simulate real-life situations where students with autism can practice social interactions, or AR can help students with dyslexia by providing interactive, 3D representations of words and letters.

- **Benefits and Challenges**: The immersive nature of AR and VR can increase engagement and motivation for students with learning disabilities. However, challenges include the cost of equipment, the need for specialized training for educators, and ensuring that content is accessible to all students.

Artificial Intelligence (AI) and Machine Learning

- **Role in Personalized Learning**: Artificial Intelligence (AI) and Machine Learning are transforming special education by enabling more personalized and adaptive learning experiences. AI can analyze student data to identify learning patterns and recommend individualized instructional strategies.

- **AI-Powered Tools**: Examples of AI-powered tools include adaptive learning platforms that adjust the difficulty of tasks based on student performance, and virtual tutors that provide personalized feedback and guidance. AI can also assist in automating administrative tasks, allowing educators to focus more on direct instruction and support.

- **Impact on Education**: AI and Machine Learning have the potential to enhance the effectiveness of special education by providing real-time insights into student progress, identifying areas where additional support is needed, and offering customized learning pathways. These technologies can help close the achievement gap for students with learning disabilities by ensuring that they receive the appropriate level of challenge and support.

Speech and Language Technologies

- **Text-to-Speech (TTS) and Speech-to-Text (STT)**: Text-to-Speech (TTS) technology converts written text into spoken words, making it easier for students with reading disabilities or visual impairments to access written content. Speech-to-Text (STT) technology, on the other hand, converts spoken language into written text, helping students with writing disabilities express their ideas.

- **Applications in Communication**: For students with severe communication impairments, speech-generating devices (SGDs) and augmentative and alternative communication (AAC) systems provide a voice, enabling them to participate in classroom activities and social interactions. These technologies can be tailored to meet the specific communication needs of each student.

- **Enhancing Learning**: Speech and language technologies empower students with learning disabilities by providing alternative ways to interact with educational content and communicate with others. They promote independence and confidence, enabling students to engage more fully in their education.

Learning Management Systems (LMS) and Educational Apps

- **Customizable Learning Platforms**: Learning Management Systems (LMS) like Google Classroom, Canvas, and Moodle are being increasingly used in special education to deliver personalized content, track student progress, and facilitate communication between educators, students, and parents. These platforms can be customized to meet the needs of students with learning disabilities, providing features like extended time for assignments, alternative formats for content, and tools for collaboration.

- **Educational Apps**: A wide range of educational apps are available to support students with learning disabilities. These apps cover various subjects and skills, from reading and math to executive functioning and social skills. Apps can provide interactive, game-like experiences that make learning more engaging and accessible.

- **Benefits and Challenges**: LMS and educational apps offer flexibility, accessibility, and the ability to tailor learning experiences to individual needs. However, it is crucial to ensure that these technologies are used effectively, with adequate training for educators and careful selection of tools that align with educational goals.

3. Integrating Techniques and Technologies in Special Education

Collaborative Approach to Implementation

- **Interdisciplinary Teams**: Effective integration of special education techniques and technologies requires collaboration among a range of professionals, including general and special education teachers, speech-language pathologists, occupational therapists, psychologists, and technology specialists. An interdisciplinary approach ensures that all aspects of the student's needs are addressed.

- **Ongoing Professional Development**: Continuous professional development is essential for educators to stay updated on the latest special education techniques and technologies. Training programs should focus on both the theoretical foundations and practical applications of these tools in the classroom.

- **Parental Involvement**: Engaging parents in the implementation process is crucial for the success of special education interventions. Parents should be informed and trained on how to use assistive technologies at home, and they should be involved in the decision-making process regarding their child's education.

Monitoring and Assessing Effectiveness

- **Data-Driven Decision Making**: The effectiveness of special education techniques and technologies should be regularly monitored through data collection and analysis. Progress monitoring tools can help educators assess whether interventions are meeting their goals and make necessary adjustments.

- **Student Feedback**: Gathering feedback from students is also important in assessing the effectiveness of interventions. Students can provide valuable insights into what is working for them and what challenges they are facing, allowing educators to tailor interventions to better meet their needs.

- **Longitudinal Studies**: Long-term studies can provide insights into the effectiveness of special education techniques and technologies over time, helping to identify best practices and areas for improvement.

4. Future Directions in Special Education

Advances in Technology

- **Emerging Innovations**: As technology continues to evolve, new tools and platforms are likely to emerge that will further enhance special education. Innovations such as brain-computer interfaces (BCIs), advanced robotics, and more sophisticated AI-driven tools could offer new ways to support students with learning disabilities.

- **Ethical Considerations**: The increasing use of technology in special education raises ethical considerations, including issues related to data privacy, equity of access, and the potential for over-reliance on technology. Educators and policymakers must carefully consider these factors as they integrate new technologies into the classroom.

Inclusive Education and Mainstreaming

- **Trends Towards Inclusion**: There is a growing trend towards inclusive education, where students with learning disabilities are integrated into general education classrooms. This approach promotes social inclusion and provides opportunities for students with disabilities to learn alongside their peers.
- **Challenges and Opportunities**: While inclusive education offers many benefits, it also presents challenges, such as ensuring that general education teachers are equipped to meet the diverse needs of their students. Technologies and techniques that support differentiation and personalized learning will be key to the success of inclusive education.

Conclusion

Special education techniques and technologies are continually evolving, offering new opportunities to enhance the learning experiences of students with learning disabilities. By leveraging evidence-based practices, innovative technologies, and collaborative approaches, educators can provide more effective support and create inclusive learning environments where all students can thrive. As the field of special education continues to advance, ongoing research, professional development, and a focus on ethical and equitable practices will be essential in ensuring that these innovations are used to their fullest potential.

Individualized Education Programs (IEPs)

Individualized Education Programs (IEPs) are foundational to special education in the United States. They ensure that students with disabilities receive tailored educational support to meet their unique needs and achieve their potential. This section provides a comprehensive overview of IEPs, covering their development, implementation, monitoring, and the key considerations for their effectiveness.

1. Overview of IEPs

Definition and Purpose

- **Definition**: An Individualized Education Program (IEP) is a legally binding document developed for each student with a disability who qualifies for special education services under the Individuals with Disabilities Education Act (IDEA). The IEP outlines the student's specific educational needs, the goals for their education, and the services and supports required to help them succeed.

- **Purpose**: The primary purpose of an IEP is to ensure that students with disabilities receive a free appropriate public education (FAPE) in the least restrictive environment. The IEP is designed to provide a customized educational plan that addresses the student's unique challenges and strengths, ensuring that they have the opportunity to make meaningful progress in their education.

Legal Framework

- **IDEA Requirements**: The Individuals with Disabilities Education Act (IDEA) mandates that IEPs be developed for all eligible students with disabilities. IDEA sets forth specific requirements for IEPs, including the components that must be included and the processes for developing, implementing, and reviewing IEPs.

- **Rights and Protections**: IDEA ensures that students with disabilities and their parents have certain rights, including the right to participate in IEP meetings, the right to be informed of decisions regarding their child's education, and the right to appeal decisions if they disagree with the IEP.

2. Components of an IEP

Present Levels of Academic Achievement and Functional

Performance

- **Current Performance**: The IEP must include a detailed description of the student's current academic achievement and functional performance. This section provides a baseline for measuring progress and helps identify areas where the student requires support.
- **Assessment Data**: Information for this section is gathered through various assessments, including standardized tests, classroom evaluations, and observations. It should reflect the student's strengths, weaknesses, and how their disability affects their ability to participate in the general education curriculum.

Measurable Annual Goals

- **Goal Setting**: The IEP must include specific, measurable annual goals that address the student's educational needs identified in the present levels of performance. Goals should be designed to help the student make meaningful progress in the general curriculum.
- **Short-Term Objectives**: For students who are not expected to achieve annual goals within a year, short-term objectives or benchmarks may be included. These provide interim targets to measure progress toward the annual goals.

Special Education and Related Services

- **Special Education Services**: The IEP must specify the special education services that the student will receive, including the type of instruction, the frequency and duration of services, and the location where services will be provided.
- **Related Services**: Related services such as speech therapy, occupational therapy, physical therapy, and counseling must also be outlined if they are necessary for the student to benefit from special education. The

IEP should detail the nature and frequency of these services.

Accommodations and Modifications

- **Accommodations**: Accommodations are changes in how instruction is delivered or how students are assessed to help them access the curriculum. Examples include extended time on tests, preferential seating, or the use of assistive technology.
- **Modifications**: Modifications are changes to the curriculum or educational standards that are designed to meet the student's individual needs. Examples include modifying the difficulty level of assignments or providing alternate forms of assessment.

Participation in General Education

- **Inclusion**: The IEP must outline the extent to which the student will participate in the general education classroom and activities. The goal is to include the student in the least restrictive environment (LRE) possible, providing access to the same educational opportunities as their peers.
- **Justification for Removal**: If the student will not participate in the general education environment, the IEP must include a justification for this decision and detail the alternative placements and supports that will be provided.

Transition Planning

- **Postsecondary Transition**: For students aged 16 and older (or younger if appropriate), the IEP must include a transition plan that outlines goals and services related to postsecondary education, vocational training, employment, and independent living.
- **Planning Components**: The transition plan should include specific goals, objectives, and activities to

prepare the student for life after high school. This may involve collaboration with vocational counselors, job coaches, and other community resources.

Measuring and Reporting Progress

- **Progress Monitoring**: The IEP must include a description of how the student's progress toward meeting their annual goals will be measured and reported to parents. This may include regular progress reports, assessments, and updates during IEP meetings.
- **Reporting to Parents**: Schools are required to provide periodic reports on the student's progress. These reports should align with the general education report cards and provide information on how well the student is meeting their IEP goals.

3. Developing and Implementing an IEP

IEP Team

- **Composition**: The IEP team typically includes the student's parents or guardians, at least one general education teacher, at least one special education teacher, a school district representative, and other individuals with knowledge or expertise relevant to the student's needs. The student may also participate in the meeting if appropriate.
- **Role of Team Members**: Each team member plays a crucial role in developing the IEP. Parents provide insights into the student's needs and strengths, teachers contribute information about academic performance and classroom behavior, and specialists offer expertise on specific areas of need.

IEP Meetings

- **Scheduling and Preparation**: IEP meetings are held at least annually but can be convened more frequently if necessary. The meeting should be scheduled at a time convenient for all participants, and parents should be provided with advance notice and an agenda.

- **Discussion and Consensus**: During the meeting, team members discuss the student's present levels of performance, set measurable goals, and decide on the appropriate services and accommodations. The goal is to reach a consensus on the IEP that reflects the student's needs and ensures a plan for their success.

Implementation and Review

- **Fidelity of Implementation**: Once the IEP is developed, it must be implemented as written. Teachers and support staff should receive training and resources to ensure they can effectively deliver the services and accommodations specified in the IEP.

- **Ongoing Review**: The IEP is reviewed at least annually to assess the student's progress, update goals, and make necessary adjustments to services or accommodations. Parents and educators should collaborate throughout the year to ensure that the IEP remains relevant and effective.

4. Challenges and Considerations

Ensuring Effective Communication

- **Between Home and School**: Effective communication between parents and educators is essential for the success of an IEP. Regular updates, meetings, and open dialogue help ensure that both parties are informed and involved in the educational process.

- **Addressing Disagreements**: Disagreements between parents and the school team may arise. It is important to address these issues through mediation or other conflict resolution strategies to ensure that the student's needs are met.

Adapting to Changing Needs

- **Updating the IEP**: As students grow and their needs change, their IEP should be updated accordingly. This may involve revising goals, changing services, or modifying accommodations to reflect the student's evolving needs.
- **Responding to New Information**: New assessments or information about the student's performance may necessitate changes to the IEP. Schools should be prepared to adjust the IEP as needed to ensure it continues to meet the student's needs effectively.

Ensuring Compliance and Quality

- **Legal Compliance**: Schools must adhere to IDEA and other relevant laws when developing and implementing IEPs. Ensuring legal compliance helps protect the rights of students with disabilities and ensures that they receive the services and supports to which they are entitled.
- **Quality Assurance**: Regular reviews of IEPs and the implementation process help maintain high-quality services for students. Schools should conduct periodic audits and evaluations to ensure that IEPs are being implemented effectively and that student progress is being monitored appropriately.

5. Future Directions for IEPs

Enhancing Family and Student Engagement

- **Increased Involvement**: Future developments in IEPs may focus on increasing family and student engagement in the planning process. This includes providing more opportunities for students to participate in goal setting and decision-making and offering additional resources and support for families.
- **Technology Integration**: Technology may play a greater role in the IEP process, with digital platforms facilitating

easier access to IEP documents, progress reports, and communication between home and school.

Focus on Holistic Development

- **Broader Goals**: There may be a shift towards incorporating broader goals in IEPs that address not only academic achievement but also social-emotional development, life skills, and career readiness.

- **Collaboration with Community Resources**: Schools may increasingly collaborate with community organizations and agencies to provide additional resources and support services that complement the educational goals outlined in the IEP.

Conclusion

Individualized Education Programs (IEPs) are a vital component of special education, providing a tailored educational plan that meets the unique needs of students with disabilities. Through careful development, implementation, and ongoing review, IEPs ensure that students receive the support necessary to succeed academically and personally. As the field of special education continues to evolve, ongoing attention to effective practices, legal requirements, and innovative approaches will be crucial in enhancing the effectiveness of IEPs and supporting the success of students with disabilities.

CHAPTER 6: HOLISTIC AND COMPLEMENTARY APPROACHES

Nutritional Influences on Learning and Behavior

Nutritional influences on learning and behavior are increasingly recognized as vital components in understanding and addressing learning disabilities. The role of nutrition in cognitive function, emotional regulation, and overall academic performance has become a significant area of research. This section explores the impact of nutrition on learning and behavior, examining key nutrients, dietary patterns, and their implications for students with learning disabilities.

1. The Role of Nutrition in Cognitive Function

Nutrients Essential for Brain Health

- **Omega-3 Fatty Acids**: Omega-3 fatty acids, particularly docosahexaenoic acid (DHA) and eicosapentaenoic acid (EPA), are critical for brain development and function. These fats are integral to the structure of neuronal membranes and are involved in neurogenesis, synaptic plasticity, and cognitive processes such as memory and attention. Studies have shown that deficiencies in omega-3 fatty acids can impair cognitive function and contribute to learning difficulties.
- **B Vitamins**: B vitamins, including B6, B12, and folate,

play a crucial role in brain health. They are involved in neurotransmitter synthesis, myelin formation, and overall brain energy metabolism. Deficiencies in these vitamins can lead to cognitive deficits, mood disorders, and impaired learning abilities.

- **Iron**: Iron is essential for oxygen transport and energy production in the brain. Iron deficiency, especially during critical periods of brain development, can lead to cognitive impairments, decreased attention span, and learning difficulties. Iron deficiency anemia is a common nutritional issue that can adversely affect cognitive performance in children.

Effects of Nutritional Deficiencies

- **Cognitive Impairments**: Deficiencies in key nutrients can result in various cognitive impairments. For example, inadequate intake of omega-3 fatty acids and iron has been linked to decreased attention, memory problems, and reduced academic performance. Identifying and addressing these deficiencies is essential for supporting optimal cognitive function.

- **Behavioral Issues**: Nutritional deficiencies can also manifest as behavioral issues, such as irritability, hyperactivity, or mood swings. These behaviors can interfere with learning and social interactions, making it important to address nutritional needs as part of a comprehensive approach to managing learning disabilities.

2. Dietary Patterns and Learning Outcomes

Balanced Diet and Cognitive Performance

- **Macronutrient Balance**: A balanced diet that includes appropriate proportions of carbohydrates, proteins, and fats supports cognitive function and overall health. Carbohydrates provide a steady supply of glucose to the brain, proteins supply essential amino acids for neurotransmitter synthesis, and fats support brain cell structure and function.

- **Meal Timing and Brain Function**: Regular meal patterns and balanced meals can enhance cognitive performance and behavioral regulation. Skipping meals or irregular eating patterns can lead to fluctuations in blood sugar levels, which may negatively impact attention and concentration.

Impact of Processed Foods and Sugars

- **Processed Foods**: Diets high in processed foods, including sugary snacks and fast food, can have adverse effects on cognitive function and behavior. These foods often lack essential nutrients and are high in unhealthy fats, sugars, and additives that may contribute to hyperactivity and poor academic performance.
- **Sugar Intake**: High sugar intake has been associated with increased risk of attention problems and hyperactivity. Excessive consumption of sugary foods and drinks can lead to fluctuations in blood sugar levels, affecting mood and cognitive performance.

3. Special Dietary Considerations for Learning Disabilities

Gluten-Free and Casein-Free Diets

- **Overview**: Some research suggests that gluten-free and casein-free diets may benefit individuals with specific learning disabilities, such as autism spectrum disorder (ASD). These diets eliminate gluten (a protein found in wheat, barley, and rye) and casein (a protein found in dairy products), which some individuals may react to adversely.
- **Evidence and Controversy**: While anecdotal reports and some studies suggest improvements in behavior and cognitive function for individuals on these diets,

the evidence is mixed. Further research is needed to determine the efficacy of these dietary interventions for learning disabilities and to identify who may benefit the most.

Micronutrient Supplementation

- **Common Supplements**: In cases where dietary intake is insufficient, micronutrient supplementation can help address deficiencies. Supplements such as multivitamins, omega-3 fatty acids, and iron may be used to support cognitive function and overall health.
- **Considerations**: Supplementation should be guided by a healthcare professional to avoid over-supplementation and to ensure that the nutrients provided are appropriate for the individual's needs. It is also important to prioritize obtaining nutrients through a balanced diet whenever possible.

4. The Influence of Hydration on Cognitive Function

Importance of Adequate Hydration

- **Cognitive Performance**: Adequate hydration is essential for optimal brain function. Dehydration can impair cognitive performance, including attention, memory, and executive function. Studies have shown that even mild dehydration can negatively impact learning and behavior.
- **Daily Hydration Needs**: Ensuring that students drink enough water throughout the day can support cognitive function and overall well-being. Schools and parents should promote regular water intake and provide access to water during the school day.

5. Strategies for Improving Nutritional Intake

Nutritional Education and Support

- **Educational Programs**: Implementing nutritional education programs for students, parents, and educators can help increase awareness of the importance of balanced nutrition and its impact on learning and behavior. These programs can provide practical tips for improving dietary habits and making healthier food choices.

- **School Meal Programs**: Schools can support students with learning disabilities by offering healthy meal options and snacks. School meal programs that emphasize fruits, vegetables, whole grains, and lean proteins can contribute to better cognitive function and behavior.

Collaboration with Healthcare Professionals

- **Nutritional Assessments**: Collaborating with dietitians or nutritionists can help identify specific nutritional needs and develop personalized dietary plans. Healthcare professionals can conduct assessments, provide recommendations, and monitor progress to ensure that students receive appropriate nutritional support.
- **Integrated Care**: Integrating nutritional support into the overall care plan for students with learning disabilities can enhance their educational outcomes. This approach involves coordinating with teachers, parents, and healthcare providers to address both educational and nutritional needs.

6. Future Directions and Research

Ongoing Research

- **Exploring New Findings**: Continued research is needed to further understand the relationship between nutrition and learning disabilities. Investigating the effects of specific nutrients, dietary patterns, and dietary interventions on cognitive function and behavior will contribute to developing evidence-based recommendations.

- **Longitudinal Studies**: Longitudinal studies can provide insights into the long-term effects of nutritional interventions on learning and behavior. These studies can help determine the effectiveness of dietary changes and inform future practices.

Personalized Nutrition

- **Individualized Approaches**: Personalized nutrition approaches that consider individual differences in metabolism, genetics, and dietary needs may offer more targeted and effective solutions for students with learning disabilities. Advances in nutritional science and technology will continue to refine these approaches.

Conclusion

Nutrition plays a critical role in influencing learning and behavior, particularly for students with learning disabilities. Ensuring adequate intake of essential nutrients, promoting balanced diets, and addressing special dietary needs can enhance cognitive function, emotional regulation, and overall academic performance. By integrating nutritional considerations into educational and healthcare practices, we can better support students with learning disabilities and help them achieve their full potential. Ongoing research and personalized approaches will further advance our understanding of the complex relationship between nutrition and learning, leading to more effective strategies for supporting students with diverse needs.

Physical Activity and Cognitive Development

Physical activity is increasingly recognized for its significant impact on cognitive development, particularly in children with learning disabilities. Regular exercise not only supports physical health but also plays a crucial role in enhancing cognitive function, improving academic performance, and promoting emotional well-being. This section explores the relationship between physical activity and cognitive development, examining mechanisms, benefits, and practical considerations for integrating physical activity into educational and therapeutic practices.

1. The Connection Between Physical Activity and Cognitive Function

Mechanisms of Cognitive Enhancement

- **Neuroplasticity**: Physical activity promotes neuroplasticity, the brain's ability to reorganize itself by forming new neural connections. Regular exercise stimulates the production of brain-derived neurotrophic factor (BDNF), a protein that supports neuron growth and synaptic plasticity. This enhancement of neural connectivity can improve cognitive functions such as memory, attention, and problem-solving.

- **Increased Blood Flow**: Exercise increases cerebral blood flow, which enhances the delivery of oxygen and nutrients to the brain. Improved blood circulation supports optimal brain function and helps maintain cognitive health. Enhanced blood flow also facilitates the removal of metabolic waste products, reducing the risk of cognitive decline.

- **Hormonal and Neurochemical Changes**: Physical activity induces the release of various hormones and neurochemicals, including endorphins, dopamine, and serotonin. These chemicals play a role in mood regulation, stress reduction, and cognitive function. Regular exercise can help stabilize mood and reduce anxiety, contributing to improved cognitive performance.

Cognitive Benefits of Physical Activity

- **Attention and Concentration**: Research has shown that physical activity can enhance attention and concentration. Exercise improves the brain's ability to focus and sustain attention, which is particularly beneficial for students with attention-deficit/hyperactivity disorder (ADHD) and other attention-related learning disabilities.

- **Memory and Learning**: Physical activity positively impacts both short-term and long-term memory. Exercise has been associated with improved verbal memory, spatial memory, and learning ability. Activities that involve complex motor skills, such as team sports, can further support cognitive processes related to learning and memory.

- **Executive Functioning**: Executive functions, including planning, organization, and impulse control, are crucial for academic success. Physical activity has been found to enhance executive functioning skills by improving cognitive flexibility, working memory, and inhibitory control.

2. Types of Physical Activity and Their Effects

Aerobic Exercise

- **Examples**: Aerobic exercises, such as running, swimming, and cycling, involve sustained physical activity that increases heart rate and breathing. These activities are known for their broad cognitive benefits and have been shown to improve overall brain health.

- **Impact**: Aerobic exercise enhances cardiovascular fitness, which in turn benefits brain function. Studies have demonstrated that regular aerobic activity can lead to improvements in cognitive performance, academic achievement, and behavioral regulation.

Strength Training

- **Examples**: Strength training exercises, including weightlifting and resistance exercises, focus on building muscle strength and endurance. These activities also contribute to cognitive health by promoting the release of growth factors that support brain function.

- **Impact**: Strength training has been associated with improved executive functions and cognitive performance. While the effects may not be as pronounced as with aerobic exercise, incorporating strength training into a well-rounded physical activity routine can provide additional cognitive benefits.

Mind-Body Exercises

- **Examples**: Mind-body exercises, such as yoga and tai chi, combine physical movement with mindfulness and relaxation techniques. These activities promote physical fitness while also enhancing mental focus and emotional regulation.
- **Impact**: Mind-body exercises have been found to improve attention, working memory, and emotional resilience. These activities can be particularly beneficial for students with learning disabilities who experience anxiety or stress, as they support both cognitive and emotional well-being.

3. Implementing Physical Activity in Educational Settings

Incorporating Physical Activity into the School Day

- **Physical Education Classes**: Schools can enhance cognitive development by offering comprehensive physical education (PE) programs that include a variety of activities, from aerobic exercises to strength training and mind-body exercises. PE classes provide structured opportunities for students to engage in physical activity and reap cognitive benefits.
- **Active Learning Environments**: Integrating physical activity into the classroom can support cognitive function and engagement. Examples include incorporating movement breaks, standing desks, and

interactive learning activities that involve physical participation.

After-School Programs and Extracurricular Activities

- **Sports and Recreation**: After-school programs and extracurricular activities, such as sports teams and recreational clubs, offer additional opportunities for physical activity. Participation in organized sports and activities can enhance cognitive skills, teamwork, and social interaction.

- **Community Programs**: Community-based physical activity programs and clubs provide further options for students to engage in regular exercise. Collaboration with community organizations can offer students access to diverse activities and support their overall development.

Individualized Physical Activity Plans

- **Tailoring Activities**: For students with learning disabilities, personalized physical activity plans can address individual needs and preferences. Working with physical educators, therapists, and parents can help design activities that are enjoyable and effective for each student.

- **Monitoring Progress**: Tracking the impact of physical activity on cognitive development and academic performance can provide valuable insights. Regular assessments and feedback can help adjust activities and ensure they are meeting the student's needs.

4. Addressing Barriers to Physical Activity

Identifying and Overcoming Obstacles

- **Accessibility Issues**: Some students may face barriers to physical activity, such as lack of access to facilities, equipment, or transportation. Schools and communities should work to address these barriers by providing accessible resources and opportunities for all students.

- **Motivation and Engagement**: Ensuring that students are motivated to participate in physical activity can be challenging. Strategies such as incorporating student interests, offering a variety of activities, and creating a supportive environment can help increase engagement.

Support and Encouragement

- **Parental Involvement**: Encouraging parents to support their children's physical activity is crucial. Providing information on the benefits of exercise and suggesting family-friendly activities can help promote a positive attitude towards physical activity at home.
- **Educator and Peer Support**: Teachers and peers play a role in fostering a supportive environment for physical activity. Positive reinforcement, encouragement, and inclusive practices can enhance students' willingness to participate in and enjoy physical activities.

5. Future Directions and Research

Exploring New Research

- **Long-Term Effects**: Future research should continue to explore the long-term effects of physical activity on cognitive development and learning outcomes. Longitudinal studies can provide insights into how sustained physical activity influences cognitive function over time.
- **Specific Populations**: Research focusing on specific populations, such as students with learning disabilities or other neurodevelopmental disorders, can help tailor physical activity interventions to meet their unique needs.

Innovations in Physical Activity Programs

- **Technology Integration**: Integrating technology, such

as fitness trackers and interactive exercise programs, can enhance physical activity interventions. Technology can provide personalized feedback, track progress, and increase engagement in physical activities.

- **Holistic Approaches**: Combining physical activity with other supportive interventions, such as nutritional guidance and behavioral therapy, can create a comprehensive approach to improving cognitive development and overall well-being.

Conclusion

Physical activity is a powerful tool for enhancing cognitive development and supporting students with learning disabilities. By promoting regular exercise, schools, families, and communities can improve cognitive function, academic performance, and emotional well-being. Implementing diverse physical activities, addressing barriers, and supporting individualized plans are essential for maximizing the benefits of physical activity. Continued research and innovative approaches will further advance our understanding of the relationship between physical activity and cognitive development, leading to more effective strategies for supporting students with learning disabilities.

Mindfulness and Stress Management

Mindfulness and stress management are emerging as crucial components in supporting the cognitive and emotional well-being of individuals with learning disabilities. The increasing recognition of the impact of psychological stress on learning and behavior underscores the importance of incorporating mindfulness practices and effective stress management techniques into educational and therapeutic frameworks. This section explores the principles of mindfulness, its benefits for cognitive development, and strategies for managing stress, particularly in the context of learning disabilities.

1. Understanding Mindfulness

Definition and Core Principles

- **Definition**: Mindfulness is the practice of focusing one's attention on the present moment with an open, accepting, and non-judgmental attitude. It involves being fully aware of one's thoughts, feelings, and bodily sensations as they occur, without attempting to change or suppress them.//
- **Core Principles**: The core principles of mindfulness include awareness, acceptance, and presence. Awareness involves recognizing and observing thoughts and feelings as they arise. Acceptance means acknowledging these experiences without judgment or resistance. Presence refers to maintaining a focused and attentive awareness of the current moment.

Mindfulness Techniques

- **Breathing Exercises**: Breathing exercises are a fundamental mindfulness technique that involves focusing on the breath to anchor attention in the present moment. Techniques such as deep breathing, diaphragmatic breathing, and mindful breathing help calm the mind and reduce stress.
- **Body Scan**: The body scan technique involves systematically focusing attention on different parts of the body to increase awareness of physical sensations. This practice helps individuals become more attuned to their bodily responses and promotes relaxation.
- **Mindful Meditation**: Mindful meditation involves sitting quietly and paying attention to thoughts, feelings, and sensations as they arise. This practice encourages non-reactive awareness and helps individuals develop a greater sense of inner calm and clarity.

2. The Impact of Mindfulness on Cognitive Function

Enhancing Attention and Focus

- **Improved Concentration**: Mindfulness practices have been shown to improve attention and concentration by training individuals to focus on the present moment. This enhanced focus can benefit students with learning disabilities who struggle with attention-related challenges.

- **Reduced Distraction**: By increasing awareness of mental processes, mindfulness helps individuals become more aware of distractions and learn to redirect their attention more effectively. This can improve academic performance and task completion.

Enhancing Memory and Learning

- **Working Memory**: Mindfulness practices have been linked to improvements in working memory, the cognitive system responsible for temporarily holding and manipulating information. Enhanced working memory can support better academic performance and problem-solving skills.

- **Information Processing**: Mindfulness may also facilitate more efficient information processing by reducing cognitive overload and improving the ability to stay focused on relevant information.

Supporting Emotional Regulation

- **Stress Reduction**: Mindfulness helps regulate emotional responses by promoting a non-reactive awareness of thoughts and feelings. This can be particularly beneficial for students with learning disabilities who experience heightened stress and emotional reactivity.

- **Resilience Building**: Through regular mindfulness practice, individuals can develop greater emotional resilience and coping skills. This enhanced resilience can support better adaptation to academic challenges and stressors.

3. Stress and Its Impact on Learning

Understanding Stress

- **Definition and Types of Stress**: Stress is a psychological and physiological response to perceived threats or demands. Stress can be acute (short-term) or chronic (long-term), and it can arise from various sources, including academic pressures, social challenges, and personal issues.
- **Stress Response**: The stress response involves physiological changes such as increased heart rate, elevated cortisol levels, and heightened alertness. While these responses can be adaptive in the short term, chronic stress can have detrimental effects on cognitive function and overall health.

Impact of Stress on Learning

- **Cognitive Performance**: Chronic stress can impair cognitive functions such as attention, memory, and executive functioning. Stress-related impairments can affect academic performance and learning outcomes, particularly for students with pre-existing learning disabilities.
- **Behavioral and Emotional Effects**: High levels of stress can lead to behavioral issues such as irritability, aggression, and withdrawal. Emotional effects include anxiety, depression, and mood swings, all of which can negatively impact a student's ability to engage in learning activities.

4. Stress Management Techniques

Cognitive-Behavioral Strategies

- **Cognitive Restructuring**: Cognitive restructuring involves identifying and challenging negative thought patterns and replacing them with more realistic and positive thoughts. This technique helps individuals manage stress by altering their perception of stressors.

- **Problem-Solving Skills**: Teaching problem-solving skills can help students approach challenges in a systematic and constructive manner. Effective problem-solving reduces feelings of helplessness and enhances coping abilities.

Relaxation Techniques

- **Progressive Muscle Relaxation**: This technique involves systematically tensing and relaxing muscle groups to reduce physical tension and promote relaxation. Progressive muscle relaxation can help alleviate stress-related physical symptoms and enhance overall well-being.
- **Visualization**: Visualization techniques involve imagining calming or positive scenarios to reduce stress and promote relaxation. Guided imagery and mental rehearsals can help students manage anxiety and improve focus.

Mindfulness-Based Stress Reduction (MBSR)

- **MBSR Program**: Mindfulness-Based Stress Reduction (MBSR) is a structured program that combines mindfulness meditation with stress reduction techniques. MBSR programs typically involve regular meditation practice, body awareness exercises, and educational components about stress and mindfulness.
- **Benefits**: MBSR has been shown to reduce stress, improve emotional regulation, and enhance overall quality of life. It can be particularly beneficial for students with learning disabilities who face high levels of academic and personal stress.

5. **Integrating Mindfulness and Stress Management in**

Educational Settings

School-Based Programs

- **Mindfulness Programs**: Implementing mindfulness programs in schools can provide students with tools to manage stress and enhance cognitive function. Programs may include mindfulness activities, meditation sessions, and stress management workshops.
- **Teacher Training**: Training teachers in mindfulness and stress management techniques can enhance their ability to support students effectively. Teachers can integrate mindfulness practices into their daily routines and provide a calming and supportive classroom environment.

Parental Involvement

- **Parent Education**: Educating parents about the benefits of mindfulness and stress management can help them support their children at home. Parents can practice mindfulness techniques with their children and create a supportive environment for managing stress.
- **Family-Based Interventions**: Family-based interventions that include mindfulness practices can promote overall family well-being and reduce stress for both parents and children. These interventions can improve family dynamics and support children's emotional and cognitive development.

Individualized Approaches

- **Tailored Interventions**: Individualized mindfulness and stress management interventions can be designed to meet the specific needs of students with learning disabilities. Personalized approaches may include one-on-one mindfulness coaching, customized stress management plans, and integration of mindfulness practices into individualized education programs (IEPs).

- **Monitoring and Evaluation**: Regular monitoring and evaluation of mindfulness and stress management interventions can help assess their effectiveness and make necessary adjustments. Collecting feedback from students, parents, and educators can provide valuable insights into the impact of these practices.

6. Future Directions and Research

Advancing Research

- **Longitudinal Studies**: Longitudinal studies are needed to explore the long-term effects of mindfulness and stress management practices on cognitive development and academic performance. Research can provide insights into the sustained benefits and optimal implementation strategies.
- **Diverse Populations**: Research should focus on diverse populations, including students with various types of learning disabilities and different cultural backgrounds. Understanding how mindfulness and stress management affect different groups can help tailor interventions to meet specific needs.

Innovations in Practice

- **Technology Integration**: Incorporating technology, such as mindfulness apps and online stress management tools, can enhance accessibility and engagement. Technology-based interventions can provide students with additional resources and support for practicing mindfulness and managing stress.
- **Holistic Approaches**: Combining mindfulness and stress management with other supportive interventions, such as physical activity and nutritional guidance, can create a comprehensive approach to enhancing cognitive and emotional well-being.

Conclusion

Mindfulness and stress management are essential components of supporting cognitive development and emotional well-being for students with learning disabilities. By incorporating mindfulness practices and effective stress management techniques into educational and therapeutic frameworks, educators, parents, and healthcare professionals can enhance students' ability to manage stress, improve cognitive function, and achieve their academic and personal goals. Continued research and innovation will further refine these practices and contribute to the development of effective strategies for supporting students with diverse needs.

Alternative Therapies: Efficacy and Evidence

Alternative therapies encompass a range of non-traditional treatments that are used alongside or instead of conventional medical and educational approaches. These therapies often focus on holistic and integrative approaches to address various aspects of health and well-being, including cognitive and emotional development. In the context of learning disabilities, alternative therapies are explored for their potential to enhance cognitive function, emotional regulation, and overall academic performance. This section evaluates the efficacy and evidence of several prominent alternative therapies, considering their application, benefits, and limitations.

1. Overview of Alternative Therapies

Definition and Scope

- **Definition**: Alternative therapies refer to practices and treatments that fall outside mainstream medical and educational approaches. These therapies often emphasize holistic and integrative methods for addressing physical, emotional, and cognitive health.
- **Scope**: The scope of alternative therapies includes a wide variety of practices such as complementary medicine, herbal remedies, acupuncture, and various forms of

bodywork and energy therapies. In the context of learning disabilities, alternative therapies are explored for their potential to support cognitive and behavioral outcomes.

2. Prominent Alternative Therapies for Learning Disabilities

Cognitive Behavioral Therapy (CBT)

- **Overview**: Cognitive Behavioral Therapy (CBT) is a structured, goal-oriented psychotherapy that focuses on identifying and changing negative thought patterns and behaviors. While traditionally used for mental health issues, CBT has been adapted to address various learning and behavioral challenges.

- **Efficacy**: Research has shown that CBT can be effective in improving executive functioning, emotional regulation, and coping strategies in individuals with learning disabilities. Studies suggest that CBT can help students develop better self-management skills, enhance problem-solving abilities, and reduce anxiety and stress related to learning challenges.

- **Evidence**: Meta-analyses and randomized controlled trials have demonstrated the efficacy of CBT in improving academic performance and reducing behavioral problems in children with learning disabilities. However, the effectiveness of CBT can vary based on individual factors and the specific nature of the learning disability.

Neurofeedback

- **Overview**: Neurofeedback is a technique that involves monitoring and providing real-time feedback on brain activity to help individuals self-regulate their cognitive and emotional states. It is used to enhance brain function and address various cognitive and behavioral issues.

- **Efficacy**: Evidence on neurofeedback for learning disabilities is mixed but promising. Some studies have indicated that neurofeedback can improve attention, cognitive control, and academic performance in individuals with ADHD and related learning challenges. However, more rigorous research is needed to establish its long-term efficacy and optimal protocols.
- **Evidence**: Systematic reviews and meta-analyses suggest that neurofeedback can have beneficial effects on attention and cognitive function, but results vary across studies. The variability in outcomes highlights the need for standardized protocols and further investigation into its effectiveness for specific learning disabilities.

Herbal Remedies and Nutritional Supplements

- **Overview**: Herbal remedies and nutritional supplements are used to support cognitive function, emotional well-being, and overall health. Common supplements include omega-3 fatty acids, Ginkgo biloba, and various vitamins and minerals.
- **Efficacy**: Research on the efficacy of herbal remedies and nutritional supplements for learning disabilities is limited but suggests potential benefits. For example, omega-3 fatty acids have been associated with improved cognitive function and reduced symptoms of ADHD. Ginkgo biloba and other herbs are sometimes used to enhance memory and cognitive performance, though evidence is less robust.
- **Evidence**: While some studies support the use of specific supplements for cognitive and behavioral improvements, the evidence is not conclusive. Variability in study design, dosage, and participant characteristics makes it challenging to draw definitive conclusions. It is important to consult healthcare

professionals before using supplements, as interactions and side effects can occur.

Acupuncture

- **Overview**: Acupuncture is a traditional Chinese medicine practice that involves inserting thin needles into specific points on the body to balance energy and promote healing. It is used to address various physical and psychological conditions.

- **Efficacy**: Research on acupuncture for learning disabilities is limited. Some studies suggest that acupuncture may help with stress reduction, mood regulation, and cognitive function. However, the evidence for its effectiveness specifically for learning disabilities is not well-established.

- **Evidence**: Systematic reviews and clinical trials have provided mixed results regarding the efficacy of acupuncture for cognitive and behavioral issues. While some studies report positive outcomes, the overall quality of evidence is low, and more research is needed to determine its effectiveness for learning disabilities.

Art and Music Therapy

- **Overview**: Art and music therapy use creative expression as a therapeutic tool to support emotional and cognitive development. These therapies involve engaging in artistic or musical activities to enhance self-expression, reduce stress, and improve cognitive function.

- **Efficacy**: Art and music therapy have been found to have positive effects on emotional regulation, social skills, and cognitive development. These therapies can provide a non-verbal means of expression and promote relaxation and creativity, which can be beneficial for students with learning disabilities.

- **Evidence**: Studies and clinical trials have shown that art and music therapy can improve various aspects of cognitive and emotional functioning. For example, music therapy has been associated with improved attention, memory, and language skills. However, the effectiveness of these therapies can vary based on individual preferences and therapy implementation.

3. Integrating Alternative Therapies into Educational and Therapeutic Practices

Holistic Approach

- **Combining Therapies**: Integrating alternative therapies with conventional approaches can provide a holistic treatment plan for students with learning disabilities. Combining therapies such as mindfulness, cognitive-behavioral strategies, and physical activity can address multiple aspects of cognitive and emotional development.
- **Individualized Plans**: Developing individualized treatment plans that incorporate alternative therapies can help meet the specific needs of students. Personalized approaches ensure that therapies are tailored to the student's strengths, challenges, and preferences.

Collaboration with Professionals

- **Multidisciplinary Teams**: Collaboration between educators, healthcare providers, and therapists is essential for effectively integrating alternative therapies into educational settings. Multidisciplinary teams can ensure that therapies are implemented appropriately and that progress is monitored.
- **Evidence-Based Practice**: Utilizing evidence-based practices when incorporating alternative therapies helps ensure that interventions are effective and

supported by research. It is important to consider the quality of evidence and the specific needs of the student when selecting therapies.

Monitoring and Evaluation

- **Assessing Outcomes**: Regular monitoring and evaluation of alternative therapies are crucial for assessing their impact on cognitive and behavioral outcomes. Tracking progress and collecting feedback from students, parents, and educators can help refine interventions and improve effectiveness.
- **Adjusting Interventions**: Based on evaluation results, interventions can be adjusted to better meet the needs of the student. Flexibility and responsiveness to individual progress and feedback are key to successful implementation.

4. Future Directions and Research

Expanding Research

- **Longitudinal Studies**: Longitudinal studies are needed to explore the long-term effects of alternative therapies on cognitive development and academic performance. Research can provide insights into the sustained benefits and potential limitations of various therapies.
- **Comparative Studies**: Comparative studies that evaluate the effectiveness of alternative therapies against traditional approaches can help identify the most effective interventions for specific learning disabilities.

Innovations and Integration

- **Innovative Approaches**: Continued innovation in alternative therapies, such as the development of new techniques and integration with technology, can enhance their effectiveness and accessibility. Exploring novel approaches can provide additional options for supporting students with learning disabilities.

- **Holistic Integration**: Integrating alternative therapies with conventional educational and therapeutic practices can create a comprehensive approach to addressing learning disabilities. Emphasizing a holistic approach ensures that all aspects of a student's well-being are considered.

Conclusion

Alternative therapies offer diverse approaches to supporting cognitive and emotional development in students with learning disabilities. While some therapies, such as cognitive-behavioral therapy and art therapy, have shown promising results, others require further research to establish their efficacy. Integrating alternative therapies with traditional approaches and tailoring interventions to individual needs can enhance overall support for students. Ongoing research, evidence-based practice, and multidisciplinary collaboration are essential for maximizing the benefits of alternative therapies and improving outcomes for students with learning disabilities.

Printed in Dunstable, United Kingdom